THE CITIZEN'S BODY

THE CITIZEN'S BODY

Desire, Health, and the Social in Victorian England

Pamela K. Gilbert

THE OHIO STATE UNIVERSITY PRESS
Columbus

Library of Congress Cataloging-in-Publication Data

Gilbert, Pamela K.
The citizen's body : desire, health, and the social in Victorian England / Pamela K. Gilbert.
p. cm.
Includes bibliographical references (p.) and index.
ISBN 978–0–8142–1052–9 (alk. paper) — ISBN 978–0–8142–9132–0 (CD-ROM) 1. Great Britain—Social conditions—19th century. 2. Public health—Great Britain—History—19th century. 3. Great Britain—History—Victoria, 1837–1901. 4. Great Britain—Civilization—19th century. I. Title.
DA533.G46 2007
942.081—dc22
2007006264

Cover design by Dan O'Dair
Text design and typesetting by Jennifer Shoffey Forsythe
Printed by Thomson-Shore, Inc.

The paper used in this publication meets the minimum requirements of the American National Standard for Information Sciences—Permanence of Paper for Printed Library Materials. ANSI Z39.48–1992.

9 8 7 6 5 4 3 2 1

CONTENTS

ACKNOWLEDGMENTS

As is usual with any project, I owe thanks to too many people to count. But here I must at least try to enumerate them, despite being doomed to the most partial of successes. Institutions first: I must mention the generous assistance and friendly atmosphere of the Wellcome Institute for the History of Medicine, and especially Sally Bragg, who makes it all function smoothly. Thanks, too, to the Wellcome Library and most especially the patient and generous Lesley Hall. The ever-reliable British Library, where I have had many happy hours, has made this book possible. Finally, the Public Records Office in Kew and the library staff at the University of Florida, especially John VanHook, all contributed to this project, as did material support from the College of Liberal Arts and Sciences and most especially the Department of English at the University of Florida.

Of my colleagues, all of whom are important sources of stimulation and support, I would like to especially thank the other Victorianists at Florida: Julian Wolfreys, Chris Snodgrass, and Alistair Duckworth. My other colleagues and friends Tace Hedrick, Susan Hegeman, Phil Wegner, Brandy Kershner, Stephanie Smith, John Murchek, Sid Dobrin, Don Ault, Kim Emery, Judith Page, Maureen Turim, Jack Perlette, Leah Rosenberg, Bernie Paris, Terry Harpold, Roger Beebe, Apollo Amoko, Marsha Bryant, Jill Ciment, Amy Ongiri, Barbara Mennell, and LaMonda Horton Stallings have given me invaluable intellectual and social nourishment. Special thanks to Patricia Craddock and Kenneth Kidd, who read and commented on earlier stages of the manuscript. Special thanks also to Malini Schueller, who read portions of the manuscript and enlightened and challenged me, helping me hone my ideas in many long conversations. Chair John Leavey's leadership and support, both intellectual and practical, have been crucial to this project; I cannot thank him enough. Of colleagues outside of Florida, I must thank especially Michael Levenson, Heidi Holder, Mark Harrison, David Wayne

Thomas, Charles Rosenberg, and Gustavo Verdesio. Thanks also to Elizabeth Langland, who has continued to be a terrific colleague and mentor, as has Jim Kincaid. Of other colleagues and correspondents, I must mention Tim Alborn, Steve Sturdy, Philippa Levine, Ryan Johnson, Susan Zieger, Yopie Prins, Martha Vicinus, Steven Mailloux, Maude Hines, Ellen McCallum, Patrick Leary, Morris Kaplan, David Pike, Rohan McWilliam, Matthew Hilton, Nancy Reisman, and many others whose comments at conferences or via e-mail have been crucial to my thinking about the larger project of which this book forms a part. Many graduate students have contributed to my thinking and helped make my intellectual environment a productive one, and I would like to thank them all but must single out Heather Milton, Michelle Sipe, and Madhura Bandyopadyay. This work or work related to it has been presented at a number of conferences and working groups, where many scholars have influenced my thinking. These include the Modern Language Association, the North American Society for Victorian Studies, the North American Conference for British Studies, various Society for the Social History of Medicine and Wellcome conferences, the Victorians' Institute, the Centre for Victorian Studies at Leeds, the Nineteenth-century and Beyond British Cultural Studies Group at the University of California Berkeley, and the Nineteenth Century Forum at the University of Michigan. Finally, I would like to thank Talia Schaffer, my other reader for The Ohio State University Press, and the two long-suffering acquisitions editors who shepherded me through the publication process, Heather Lee Miller and Sandy Crooms.

Clare Ford Wille, Peter Shahbenderian, and Daniel Kirkpatrick, excellent friends and fountains of knowledge and kindness, have supported my work unreservedly for the seemingly endless series of summer research visits it has taken to see it completed. I would like, finally, to thank family and friends Angela Geitner, Meryl Strichartz, Nicolet de Rose, Tace Hedrick, and Kenneth Kidd for laughter, love, conversation, and perspective.

INTRODUCTION

Society has conquered the public realm.
—Hannah Arendt

In 1958 Hannah Arendt looked back over the troubled history of late modernity—the rise of democracy and of fascism, of the extension of citizenship and of semipermanent states of exception—and penned *The Human Condition,* her analysis of our political heritage and its possible futures. Early in the volume she devotes considerable space to the rise of the social, a historical fact she regards with resigned bitterness. According to Arendt, when late modernity, with its large populations organized into nation-states, enabled the realm of the household to invade the political arena, the social was born—and promptly, like the cuckoo in the nest, the social destroyed the legitimate existing domains of public and private upon which all truly political action could be based. What remains of the extinct demos is a mass of people without individuality who have lost the capacity to act and can now only "behave."

In 1962 Jürgen Habermas would cover some of the same ground in *The Structural Transformation of the Public Sphere,* at least somewhat more optimistically. During the same period when Arendt sees the political suffocating under the weight of the social, Habermas sees the birth of a vibrant public sphere. Despite the fact that this early work traces a rather dire debilitation of that public sphere in later years, Habermas's oeuvre argues for a fairly optimistic vision of a new kind of political participation that emerges in this period, through the public sphere. Even if incompletely realized, he argues, this public of rational debate between putative equals allows for a new political relationship between an empowered public and sovereignty, which he sees as the ultimately worthwhile goal of the Enlightenment project. He, too, however, sees peril to this ideal from the intrusion of "private matters"—

identity issues, for example—in the public sphere. In this, at least, he agrees with Arendt's sense of the dangers of the introduction of the private into matters of state.

However, the growth of the public sphere that Habermas celebrates and the emergence of the social that Arendt decries are not discrete events. It is, I will argue, the social as a mediating domain that enables the development, in this transitional period, of a notion of liberal government that can mediate between "matters of the household" and those of citizenship, both allowing for and policing a more inclusive model of political participation.[1] Far from destroying the public and private, the social permits the development of a specifically modern understanding of public and private, in which the structurally necessary fantasy of a public-private divide can be sustained through the reformulation of older models of citizenship. In allowing "matters of the household"—of the body and the realm of necessity—into public discourse about the social body, the realm of the social provided a way to connect the management of individual bodies to citizenship, while still allowing "private matters" to remain outside the boundaries of politics per se. Although perhaps ultimately untenable, this double gesture—of making the private central to government while apparently excluding it from political representation—allows modern liberal government to develop and function in a complex and changing period.

This volume thus addresses a fundamental problem in Victorian notions of citizenship—a problem that remains thorny for liberal theorists today. What is the role of the social in creating and sustaining the ideals of national

1. A word is in order here about the use of the term "liberal," which I use not in the specific sense of the Liberal Party (except when capitalized) or of a particular political theory. There were many kinds of liberals, of course, in mid-Victorian society, espousing theories from the economic liberalism of Smith to that of the later Mills, which emphasized social responsibility while retaining a largely Kantian notion of a core individual self. But I am referring here to the overarching philosophy of government in the period, stemming from Enlightenment ideals and largely shared by Tories and Whigs, and later by Conservatives, Liberals, and most Radicals alike. These ideals include the conviction that government should in some sense be representative, interest itself in building the good society (or in removing impediments to its development), be based when feasible on consent rather than force, and be founded on the inviolability of property and a relatively free circulation of labor, capital, and goods. It is at base a capitalist and possessive individualist vision. Although there were different interpretations of core terms, this was generally the ideal of government that most Victorians shared, and the one that comes under the broad term "liberal." Thus, many people identified economic and social policies as "liberal," especially in the beginning of the period, that we might see as conservative today because they were based on a fundamentalist view of economic liberalism. By the time the "Liberal" Party came along, the term had come to be associated with social policies favoring the extension of the franchise as later it would be connected to "social" measures such as universal education. But I am using the term here in its most catholic sense, and in that sense, Victorian Britain was marked by a steadily liberalizing vision of government.

community? How does the private self relate to the public one? And how can freedom of choice work to uphold a common ideal in a society in which cultural and personal values seem unmanageably diverse? As the idea of citizenship grew to be more inclusive, and liberalism posited a society of eventual universal citizenship, England confronted the problem of those whose behaviors did not seem to indicate fitness for the responsibilities associated with political power. In a liberal society, fit behaviors had to originate in individual choices rather than in coercion from above. In a market economy, rewards were held to accrue to those behaviors that were socially appropriate. Yet what of those who did not choose to behave appropriately? What of those who disregarded such rewards? Political economists and their early popularizers, such as Harriet Martineau, tended to assume that such misbehaviors (early marriages, bad saving habits, etc.) were the result of ignorance. Because establishing financial security, increasing social status, and nurturing a family were increasingly held to be natural human desires, those who failed to behave in ways designed to achieve those goals were assumed to be ill-informed. Once people understood the laws of economics, it was reasoned, they would certainly begin to behave appropriately, engaging in a kind of social citizenship that might (or might not) be the precursor of a suffrage-based citizenship.

By the mid-century it had become evident that this had been a utopian belief. Behaviors were based not on the intellectual awareness of enlightened self-interest but on the desire for the good things that those behaviors could bring. And too many people displayed desires that were antithetical to the notion of fitness championed by liberal thinkers. Thus, social outreach became a matter not simply of giving information but of a more comprehensive education leading to the management of desire, which in turn required an active role in the very formation of subjectivity. Since these desires were supposed to be natural, they were rooted in the private sphere—in the body and the family, believed to be the natural, universal substrata of the individual and social units. Preparation for citizenship came to be seen less as a matter of acquiring a public and political identity than of shaping the familial, moral, and physical environment required to foster a natural and healthy body and mind; in short, with liberal universalism, fitness for citizenship ceased to be simply a political issue and became instead explicitly a social matter rooted in the private and domestic spheres. The management of the social body through public medicine and discourses of health became the principal discourse with which to negotiate these new questions of citizenship and the Condition of England, of the fit individual and the problematic masses. The development of this discourse identified the healthy body and healthy desires as the basis of political fitness. Over the course of this period, the citizen became not only a moral product of education but also a physical product of good domestic hygiene.

A flurry of recent books on Victorian liberalism focus on anxieties surrounding the figure of the citizen. Richard Dellamora's *Friendship's Bonds* traces the ideal of male homosocial bonds within a "just society . . . governed by friends" (1) and its shadow, anxieties about male homosexual exploitation—the fear that the city on a hill would become the cities of the plains. Amanda Anderson's *The Powers of Distance* also examines problematic figures of liberal anticitizenship (and antimodernity). The celebrated powers of reason and cosmopolitan detachment valued by liberalism led to fears that such detachment taken to extremes undoes liberalism itself—taking the citizen toward rootlessness, dandyism, dilettantism, and amoral sensation-seeking. Anderson traces the anxiety around detachment specifically through aesthetic debates of the period. David Wayne Thomas's *Cultivating Victorians* also examines the ideal of liberal agency in relation to aesthetic value; his concern centers more on questions of authenticity and the staging of the self through various cultural debates. Finally, Lauren Goodlad's splendid *Victorian Literature and the Victorian State* is most closely related to the concerns of this book, as it focuses on the oscillation between the desire for a managerial state and one fostering autonomy, a model of state as pastor. All of these studies focus on the anxieties of liberalism—in an inclusive state, what are the limits of inclusion? When does the nation itself lose its identity, and on what is that identity based? They also all identify nodes of anxiety around questions of individual agency and autonomy.

This book intersects with these recent works in a variety of ways. Anderson and Thomas attempt a revalorization of liberal values and frequently make compelling arguments to support their positions—among them, critiques of the tendency of recent scholarship to reject such values wholesale. Although sympathetic to many of the core values of liberalism that these authors advance, I attempt in this volume to provide a balanced critique of the problems and contradictions within those values, as well as the opportunities those contradictions have historically created. In the works above, also, whether citizenship is articulated through aesthetic practices, practices of consumption, sexual practices, or anxieties about identity, these debates tend to be articulated through ideals of normalcy—the normal individual's tastes and practices in relationship to the "healthy" ideal self or the deviant other. Rather than focusing primarily on those tastes and practices, however, this book focuses also on the ground of those tastes: the body. This book traces the construction of citizenship through the figure of the healthy body, in parliamentary debates on the franchise, in sanitary and housing publications, and in novels. Throughout the mid-century, evolving discussions of the healthy body and its tastes would undergird debates about individuality, the social body, and fitness for citizenship.

Much scholarship on the Victorian period in the past several years, following the insights of Foucault, has addressed the social body, a key term for the same period, and its relationship to the state. The rise of liberal government and new knowledge directed at measuring and controlling the economic and physical behaviors of the populace have a strong relationship to Victorian ideas about fitness and citizenship. Yet little work has explicitly connected these two areas of scholarship.[2] In Victorian Britain the discussion of the franchise developed in the context of industrial capitalism and a slow enlargement of the polis, which allowed for a protracted and richly complex debate on the formation of the fit citizen and citizenship's relationship to class and gender identity. In this period the legislative and cultural basis developed, not only for a modern liberal notion of citizenship as defined by political rights but also for its social corollaries. The emergence of the social as a key domain is fundamental to the definition of public and private that materializes over the long and troubled period marked by the First and Second Reform Bills (1832 and 1867). Yet this social sphere, of which much has been said, has actually been ill-defined in scholarly discussion. Theorists such as Mary Poovey, Jacques Donzelot, and Patrick Joyce have each placed its origination in historical periods more than one hundred years apart, a discrepancy that has not been adequately addressed. Finally, the operations of the social in relation to articulations of public and private have not been fully explained.

As a metaphorical description of a population in corporeal terms, the "social body" had a long history in the early modern period and took on renewed importance in the late eighteenth and early nineteenth centuries, as discussions of the social body coincided with new views of the state's role as a manager of physical health and facilitator of social cohesion. The social body should not be confused with earlier and very different concepts, such as the monarch's two bodies, or the public, or the state. The "body of the people" is probably the closest concept. But only in the late eighteenth century did

2. A notable exception is Patricia McKee's fine analysis of the gendered knowledge systems operating through the public-private divide in the late eighteenth and nineteenth centuries.

a concept emerge of a body of the nation that was neither identical with the politically active portion of the population nor simply the economic one. This new understanding of the body of the people positioned it as one to be managed in terms of its health, reproduction, and morality. This body was constitutive of the state but still disconnected from direct political influence. In the early nineteenth century, as political representation became conceptually linked to the social body for the first time (with the threat and promise of an ever-expanding suffrage), the social body began also to be medicalized. As Foucault's work emphasizes, with the advent of new statistical practices to analyze the population, the figure of the social body as understood in this period divided society into masses of standardized or deviant individual bodies.[3] Vice came to be seen less as the result of fallen nature than as the perversion of nature through adverse circumstances, such as living in urban poverty. Moral health was understood as coterminous with physical health; political normalcy was dependent on this healthy state. The advent of epidemic disease in urban areas lent both focus and urgency to this understanding of the social body. It also provided it with a vocabulary founded on the notion of physically healthy bodies as the basis of the modern state. Healthy subjects—structurally equivalent and behaviorally similar—would behave rationally and appropriately; hence, statistical science would not only measure but also predict behavior, contributing to the transparency of a thoroughly modern society. As the century wore on, this model was inflected with a number of other ways of reading the healthy body, including ethnicity (especially as compared to the Irish in the 1830s, 1840s, and 1850s) and emerging modern notions of race (mostly from the mid-1850s on). But these ways of reading "deviance" largely participated in and built on the sanitary rhetoric established earlier, as Irish or Indian bodies were read as "naturally" dirty or prolific.[4]

3. Some readers may be surprised to find Foucauldian and Habermasian scholars side by side in this volume. Poovey's analysis of the making of the social body is fundamental for me, and I see my work here in part as extending her analysis. Habermas and Nancy Armstrong have also provided me with key insights for understanding the period. Although I have fundamental differences with Habermasian liberalism, his work as a historian is foundational. Some historians have critiqued *Structural Transformation* as overgeneralizing and idealizing a never-never coffee house culture that did not live up to its own notion of itself. But Habermas is here a historian of an ideal; that is, he gives us a clear history of what people hoped for and believed in, if not of actual practices. That ideal is, of course, still very much with us. Foucault gives us a somewhat more cynical history of the epistemologies associated with those developments. In this sense, the two projects are complementary.

4. The impact of empire on visions of citizenship and the body cannot be underestimated, and clearly, the Irish famine, the Jamaica uprisings, and the Indian Rebellion of 1857 all weighed heavily on British visions of the nation and the body, although it is beyond the scope of this study to treat these topics with the care they deserve. For a discussion of the impact of empire on British understandings of public health at home, see Gilbert, *Mapping the Victorian Social Body*.

In the reform debates that took place between 1832 and 1867, the concept of citizenship was elaborated in relation to the franchise, which made elite perception of the working classes the site of contention about what constituted a right to or fitness for participation in government. The sense of fitness that developed, although formally tied to economic requirements, was increasingly defined in social terms. The first reform shifted qualification from property ownership to levels of consumption. Additionally, by the 1860s the criterion of "fitness" as a qualification to exercise the vote came to predominate; key to fitness was "individuality." At the same time, in both political and sanitary rhetoric, the "masses" were seen as the antithesis of individuality and citizenship. The "fit" working man was by the 1860s defined as he who was able to act as an individual, defined in part by his modes of consumption, rather than as a part of a mass; the unfit noncitizen—the pauper, for example—was part of an aggregate who lacked individual interests and the ability to reason. This fear of the realm of necessity—of the body—reflects what J. G. A. Pocock calls an Aristotelian strand in Victorian theories of liberal citizenship: those caught within the realms of necessity, too engaged with bodily needs, were seen as requiring socialization before emerging into the public sphere, which was carefully separated from the domestic. This division perpetuated an illusion of politics as separable from materiality and economics, and of a bourgeois individual self that preceded the "mass" of humanity and was separate from it.

The social body, then, includes and depends upon a definition of the (ideal) body of the individual citizen. "Citizenship" is constructed as dependent on the internalization of certain kinds of desire and their enactment as consumption of goods and services (especially housing) and information. Thus, to make the pauper into a good citizen, it is necessary to teach him or her to desire appropriately—usually framed as desire for marriage, financial security, and upward mobility for one's family. Citizenship, although defined as public and male, is therefore dependent on the domestic sphere—that is, on private and female modes of production and reproduction. Not surprisingly then, anxiety about the control of the working classes is centered on (feminine or feminized) inappropriate desires and on the inappropriate desires of middle-class women.

"Citizenship" is connected to the rise of the national narrative and positions itself explicitly as a category of identity overriding class identification; it is constructed to operate as a counter to class politics by incorporating all classes within a shared civic culture of appropriate consumption. Every citizen is a citizen of something. If not members of a class or other identity group, individuals could not simply be monads, floating free of all communal sentiment. The imagined community that legitimated citizenship was the nation. National identity, as a widely shared identity value, comes into sharp focus in this period precisely as public authority is contested and as other identities, such as class, begin to appear threatening as loci of power. As Habermas's analysis suggests, it required the presence of a public sphere, within which narratives of national identity might be played out in relationship to the concept of individual, private (bourgeois) identity being formulated in the novel. Western liberal notions of citizenship rely on this divide to safeguard both individual freedom and a state that is putatively free of identity politics. This division has, of course, been extensively critiqued as an ultimately untenable, if strategically necessary, fiction. Though national identity is fundamentally a *public* identity, it is one of the peculiar markers of this period and its rhetoric that individuals internalized their sense of this public self as a fundamental, physical (and later, racial) essence, which nonetheless never fully lost the public character bound up in the concept of citizenship.

As sanitarians struggled to extend their legal influence, the discourse of moral environmentalism contributed to the conception of healthful environment as a prerequisite of citizenship; health, like literacy, was something to which the potential citizen must have access. Health was defined as a set of hygienic practices that created a bodily habitus appropriate to the development of middle-class tastes, thus eradicating class boundaries. It was necessary to the nation that workers be both healthy and fit citizens, rather than physically degenerate and politically disaffected—either apolitical or, worse, identifying primarily with class interests. Paradoxically, then, the desire to separate the political man—self-as-citizen—from the realm of the body and necessity demanded an increasingly anxious emphasis on the body itself. The notion of the social body became a way to talk about the connection between the public sphere of nation and the private sphere of individuals, while citizenship—both as a way of defining the person as a member of the national social body and as the institutional link between nation and state—became the measure and the goal of its health.

Thus, national identity, as it operated in the mid-nineteenth century, was beginning to be defined in the public sphere as a link between the individual and the population as a whole—in short, as a mode of interpellation of the citizen, the public identity of the private man. The complete match between the nation and the social body could only be achieved if all members could be brought within that narrative and made into good, healthy citizens who identified with the nation as an overarching category more fundamental than other identities, especially class. Many institutions contribute to this process, but perhaps none so fundamentally as that state-supported but private ideological apparatus, the family. Liberal inclusiveness demanded the careful and untiring construction of a subject perfectly free to act in accordance with his or her desires, provided those desires were "natural"—that is, constructed within increasingly narrow definitions of the normal and appropriate. Most of these desires had to do with domestic, "private" life and the reproduction of the family in a bourgeois mode.

Thus Britishness equals Englishness equals, by the end of the period, the healthy (clean, isolated), white, masculine, middle-class body. Women became the privileged site of production of this body through their ability to construct an appropriately domestic environment. As Foucault has argued, the move toward modern liberal government is marked by "governmentalities"—the development of bodies of knowledge that are also practices, particularly in regard to biopolitics (the management of populations) through public health, the census, and the like, which enabled governments to know about both the movements and living habits of their subjects. This information was also used to mobilize consent among those subjects to governmental aims, rather than relying on brute power. The discourses and practices that emerged in Britain in regard to these developments authorized themselves with the rhetoric of national identity, interest, and improvement; those we will engage include some of those associated with the development of the sanitary and housing movements and their relation to the emerging concept of the social body, especially in combination with citizenship and the franchise, domesticity, and pauperism.

What would come to be understood over the course of the period as public health—especially in relation to epidemic disease and sanitary issues—has a privileged role in the discourses of the social body. The public health debate did much to foreground the body and its environment as the basis of national health and morality; as the body took center stage in these discourses, citizenship itself came to be perceived as having a physical basis. The body itself is a key signifier. Basic representative of a materiality that is malleable yet limited, the body became in this period both the index and the metaphor of the nation. Individual bodies and their ills, as representatives of classes and populations, became indices of the condition of that less tangible entity, the social body; early on, the social itself, in both its physical and its moral manifestations, came to be understood as a medicalized physical entity that could be fixed, observed, and dissected both through the individual bodies of its subjects and in toto (or en masse) in the form of statistics. The social, like a body (and like the economy), was supposed to work according to "natural laws," laws that, nevertheless, had to be carefully learned. Because of this formulation, the social was not considered amenable to legislative or political solutions, but it was to pedagogical ones, especially those situated in the home.

This volume traces the discourse on the citizen and the social body in three forms of discourse in the public sphere. Section I of this book focuses on mid-nineteenth-century political views of citizenship. The first two chapters of this section provide a detailed analysis of parliamentary debates on the franchise and an exposition of competing notions of political fitness. Within these debates we can also trace the impact of sanitary visions of the body—connected to English political discourse partly through the aleatory conjunction of a major cholera epidemic arriving concurrently with reform agitation—on notions of political fitness for citizenship. Social issues coalesced around sanitary questions, just as political enfranchisement was insistently connected to the health of the social body. By the mid-century, as we see in chapter 3, progressive politics came to be allied with sanitary intervention. Victorians thus set the stage for a time when health, like education, would be a right of the nascent citizen; however, Victorian liberalism's mystification of the interdependence of the political, social, domestic, and economic would also retard the recognition of those rights and contribute to their erosion in the latter years of the twentieth century.

Section II focuses on the social. In these three chapters, we shall examine how interventions in the domain of the social—specifically in the housing movement—clarify the relationship between the political, economic, domestic, and sanitary projects of the mid-Victorian period. First, chapter 4 offers a careful theorization of the divisions between public, private, and the social that clarifies the stakes of the succeeding readings. The well-wrought individual was thought to emerge from a physical environment that would foster not only health but also suitable values. It was in the domestic sphere that these values were formed. For this reason, following earlier successes at sanitizing the city, social outreach turned to the domestic environment. Yet the social need to house the poor well conflicted with the economic doctrine that charity pauperized by undermining independence. Chapter 5 explores the mid-century emphasis on inculcating bourgeois norms of privacy and separation in multiroom dwellings and how it conflicted with the reality of high urban rents and the habits of city-dwelling laborers. These and other problems encouraged social reformers to look not only at the built environment but also at the behaviors and the desires of the poor. The poor, it was concluded, were problematic because of structural and economic problems and because their desires, shaped by their unusual home lives, were warped. Social workers, then, needed to address not only the physical environment but also the unhealthy desire that it produced and reflected.

Because it dealt with this feminized domain of the home and the body, social intervention offered special opportunities for middle-class women. Yet as the social became central to the national project, it called increasingly for a professionalized class of social workers. Such professionalization threatened the status of the social as an autonomous domain emerging from the private by bringing it under state control. In chapter 6 Octavia Hill provides a transitional example: as the last representative of the mid-Victorian concept of liberal social action, she espoused a vision that tended inevitably toward the more professionalized activism of the 1880s and 1890s while highlighting, by her resolute refusal to acknowledge that trend, the particular issues of the mid-Victorian vision of the social. Her work is revelatory of the roots of difficulties still with us today (especially in the United States), in terms of both wedding social activism to liberal democracy and reclaiming a tradition of female activism rooted in the separation of the social from political action. This history is particularly problematic for feminism, as the separation of the social is in part based on the discourse of the social as a body and the cultural associations of the body with a feminized system of care and a discourse of "nature" that is separate from culture and politics.

Section III turns to the novel and, with it, to the representation of the individual. Hannah Arendt called the novel of the late eighteenth and nineteenth centuries "the only entirely social art form" (39). The novel is the privileged forum for the exploration and celebration of middle-class Victorian subjectivity and domesticity, as well as one of the most important arenas for social commentary in this period. In chapter 7 the mid-century "social problem" novel enables us to examine narratives of the development of the social, sanitary reform, and their relation to the political in works by Benjamin Disraeli and Margaret Oliphant. After the initial flurry of Condition of England novels and the failure of the Charter, social fitness came to be defined less explicitly in terms of the franchise and more in terms of individual development. The fit body was defined in terms of continence and incontinence, and the fit subject was marked by a painfully achieved moral and physical self-containment, as we will see elaborated in Elizabeth Gaskell and Charles Dickens in chapter 8. Finally, George Eliot's *Felix Holt* rereads mid-century social problem novels in consideration of this attention to moral hygiene. Chapter 9 demonstrates how Eliot recuperates and revises an earlier tradition in both political writing and sensation novels in using addiction as a thematic correlative for politically unfit behaviors. The closed, disciplined bourgeois body requires careful development and policing and is always under the threat of invasion and dissolution through mismanagement of its own desires. Intemperance and addiction become dominant themes for thinking through the threats to civic "fitness" in these novels, just as the beneficent influence of the feminized social is expressed through plotlines that emphasize sanitary reform and social work.

Thus, the book examines the epistemology of cultural divisions into public, private, and social domains and links the development of these concepts to the problems of class, gender, and citizenship that are particularly volatile in the mid-Victorian period. The striking centrality of medical discourse to politics and government in the context of parliamentary reform, women's social activism, and conceptions of English identity testify to the importance of the body and ideas of health to citizenship. In each of the three sections of the book, a different kind of discourse is examined. At the state level, parliamentary debates lay out an explicitly political agenda for citizenship. These debates concern not only ideological questions but also structural ones—how will the newly enfranchised affect the existing system? Sanitary writings also deal with questions of the moral and physical health of the public and are written to encourage political change—that is, changes in legislation and policy. In the second section, social experts in the field of housing are largely writing to each other and to the general public. This shift not only reflects the reification of social intervention, in that it constitutes particular and specialized fields such as housing, which are public issues without being state issues per se, but also its general importance throughout the culture, as charity is systematized and organized under social theories. Such documents, generally intended to be persuasive to a general public, appeal to broadly understood notions of social appropriateness and desirable behavior in the service of specific arguments. The final section examines the incorporation of such narratives into novels, emphasizing the centrality of public health and its formulations of the social in the liberal domestic novel of the mid-century. These novels, like the texts explored in earlier sections, seek to communicate with the general public on political or social questions. But with their focus on private life and the elaboration of private subjectivities, they also offer detailed explorations of the relation between narratives of public and private life unavailable in the other discursive arenas studied here. In this section we can trace the increasing centrality of constructions of bodily desire and continence to these narratives over the course of the mid-century.

Each group of writings addresses fitness for citizenship in a different way, with different audiences and emphasis. Yet all, finally, concern the body, its environment, and its desires. The notion of the medicalized social body emerges as the most significant way to mediate competing discourses of citizenship and nationhood, of the individual and the larger community. The development of the discourses explored here foregrounded the healthy body as the very basis of political fitness and defined the condition of England in terms of individual healthy bodies and the management of desire to produce the ideal bodily habitus. From the first reform seen as a potential cause of national ills to a second reform positioned as an inadequate cure for national incontinence, we can trace the establishment of a self-contained English body as a *sine qua non* of citizenship and the definition and disciplining of the social as its nurturing medium.

SECTION I

Citizenship and the Social Body

1

CITIZENSHIP AND FITNESS

> If you want venality, if you want ignorance, if you want drunkenness, and facility for being intimidated; or if, on the other hand, you want impulsive, unreflecting and violent people, where do you look for them in the constituencies? Do you go to the top or to the bottom? . . . We know what those persons are who live in small houses . . . and no better law, I think, could have been passed than that which disfranchised them altogether.
>
> —Robert Lowe, MP

> Whether we take education in schools; whether we take social conduct; whether we take obedience to the law; whether we take self-command and power of endurance, shown under difficulty and privation; whether we take avidity for knowledge and self-improvement—if we apply any of these tests, or any other test that can be named . . . if the working man in some degree was fit to share in political privileges in 1832 he has, at any rate, attained some degree of additional fitness now.
>
> —William Ewart Gladstone, Chancellor of the Exchequer, 1866

What did it mean to talk about fitness for the franchise in this period? In this chapter I would like to briefly examine competing models of citizenship during the period in question and trace the emergence of the important theme of individualism versus the masses in citizenship debates from the 1830s to the 1860s. The concept of the individualized voter that came to dominate the understanding of fitness in the 1860s crystallized around two questions: How could the worker, trapped in the realm of necessity, develop the kind of independent understanding of issues that would qualify him for the vote? And what was the role of potential mediating identities such as class in the worker's ability to act as an individual? For many Victorian commentators, the nightmare of corporative political action based on class was imaged in terms of the massed bodies of the poor.

Models of Citizenship

Citizenship, as we, the heirs of a complex liberal tradition, now conceive it, requires at minimum a recognition of the individual's right (and duty) to participate in government. An implicit part of citizenship is the right of the person to an environment and resources that foster the abilities necessary for citizenship and—much less clearly and more recently—some sense of a corresponding duty of the state to provide those conditions. British sociologist and policy analyst T. H. Marshall famously contended that this concept of citizenship requires the simultaneous existence of three levels of rights: civil, political, and social, which have developed in the modern world at different rates. In the mid-Victorian period, he asserts, civil rights were basically in place, and political rights were being hammered out, most conspicuously in the two major reform bills. Social rights, however, were "in the doldrums." Even as the first major reform bill was passed in 1832, just two years later, Marshall argues, the passage of the New Poor Law in 1834 was a decisive defeat of social rights: "the minimal social rights that remained were detached from the status of citizenship. The Poor Law treated the claims of the poor, not as an integral part of the rights of the citizen, but as an alternative to them—as claims that could be met only if the claimants ceased to be citizens," noting that paupers forfeited both "personal liberty . . . and . . . any political rights they might possess" (Marshall and Bottomore, 15).

Strikingly, however, Marshall concludes that the one social right that did develop in the nineteenth century was education—"a personal right combined with a public duty to exercise the right . . . because the social health of a society depended on the civilisation of its members." In this way the state recognized that "its culture is an organic unity and its civilisation a national heritage" (ibid., 16). In short, the one social right that did develop was that which provided a minimal level of opportunity for the development of abilities, in children, necessary for the future exercise of citizenship, defined as identification with a national, rather than local, identity.[1] This

1. Children are of particular interest within liberalism because they represent the limit case of individual freedom and responsibility. An adult, according to economic liberalism, has the choice to work or starve, to participate in the political process or ignore it, to opt in or out of the system. But a child does not—nor can the child, if she or he grows to adulthood without minimal skills required for participation in society (literacy, for example), choose freely even after attaining adulthood. Children are potentially free, but they exist in a state of unfreedom and dependency that affects that potential. Therefore, in theory, children—and laborers were often described as moral and political children in this period—enjoin particular responsibilities on the liberal state (which can be conceived of as the children's rights), despite having yet no corresponding responsibilities of their own. Over the course of the nineteenth century, as health was seen as a minimal prerequisite of citizenship, the child's health came to be something of a political issue, despite its dependence on factors traditionally outside the political domain—the parents' work habits, for example, or domestic circumstances.

shows that the social domain was already identified as an important fostering ground for fitness, even if its status as a domain implying rights was still nascent.

But there is no doubt that in the nineteenth century inclusion in the nation was increasingly formulated in political terms, as opposed to earlier concepts of "the people" based on passive inclusion in a territorial definition of the state. The political rights that form part of the basis of modern citizenship developed in the nineteenth century through the extension of the franchise. That process made the working classes the site of a debate by elites (here defined broadly as members of groups with political and hegemonic authority) on what constituted fitness for participation in government. An uneasy relationship between the understanding of working men as individuals and as representatives of a class emerges over the period of 1832–67, bounded by the first two reform bills. Here I would like to examine the development of a notion of individualist citizenship as set against the category of social class as a "massing" function, in relation to reform, especially in the 1860s. I will then explore some of citizenship's connections to the sanitary movement and the construction of the healthy body. This body depended on a habitus promoting middle-class habits of consumption,[2] and this physical "fitness" was intimately connected to political fitness for the franchise.

During the period on which we will focus, two reform bills passed, one in 1832 and one in 1867. These were not the last reforms, but they were among the most significant. The First Reform Bill passed amidst a flurry of rioting and the threat of revolution. It focused on the elimination of rotten boroughs and enfranchisement of newly powerful and populous urban areas, on the elimination of certain kinds of bribery and political corruption, and on the extension of the vote to an emerging class of respectable but not heavily propertied men. It is this last change with which we will be most concerned. It extended the electorate in a way that, though not as numerically significant as many reformers had hoped, allowed for a complete revision of the very basis of the right to vote. The second reform was much less dramatic, though it extended the franchise to a fairly large class of people (nearly doubling the electorate); in the end it was quite a conservative measure that, by offering the illusion of substantive reform, stemmed the demand for working-class representation for a few more years. Universal male suffrage would not take

2. I use the term "habitus" in the sense in which Pierre Bourdieu uses it—as a revision of the Aristotelian notion of *hexis,* a learned moral character that becomes constitutive of the subject's desires. Bourdieu modifies it to account for the structural (here, classed) character of *hexis,* so that the emphasis is reciprocally and equally on individual subjectivity and on the generative power of social structures that precedes the individual (see *Outline of a Theory of Practice*, 261 and passim). Habitus is phenomenologically grounded in the individual's sense of his or her body.

place until 1918, let alone universal adult suffrage, which was legislated in 1928. However, this second reform is significant because it marks an overt engagement with notions of fitness connected to the social sphere that would form the foundation of the more socially and politically radical period that would follow it. It marks the culmination and end of the high Victorian period.

In the 1832 reform debates there was little talk of a right to the franchise. Instead, the debates were dominated by a combination of topics: the threat of revolution, concern for balance of representation (i.e., worry that elites would be overwhelmed by the new constituencies), and talk of the "ten pounders'" (that is, the occupant of property worth at least ten pounds per annum) increasing fitness to use such power responsibly. The closest allusion to a "right" was in talk of a "natural desire" in an educated and increasingly propertied population to participate in government. Although the appeal to "nature" sets us on the road to a liberal perception of a right—after all, what is natural must be appropriate, and what is appropriate must be just—this is still a long way from a right of citizenship or an obligation of the state. Fitness thus implied ability, but ability implied no corresponding right yet, only a corresponding desire.[3]

The 1860s, unlike the 1830s or even the 1840s and 1850s, saw little direct threat of violence in the pursuit of political rights.[4] The reform debates, taken up again in the late 1850s and early 1860s after the defeat of Chartism and of Lord John Russell's bill in 1854 (Russell was a long-term reform advocate),[5] continued, in effect, for seven years. This leisurely discussion afforded the time for a meticulous untangling (and retangling) of the difficult question of inclusion in the social body. No longer having recourse to the driving fear of revolution, proreform MPs,[6] most often affiliated with the Liberal Party in

3. According to Frank O'Gorman, the electorate increased from about 14 percent of all adult males to 18 percent after1832. Between the two reform bills, the proportion remained steady. By 1868, 54 percent of adult males (12 percent of the population) had the franchise (182). For a full discussion, see O'Gorman, *Voters, Patrons, and Parties.*

4. I except here the Hyde Park "riots," because they occurred only after the reform bill was defeated in 1866. Following this defeat, there were (mostly peaceful) demonstrations all over the country. However, in late July the Reform League marched to Hyde Park to hold a public meeting. The home secretary ordered the gates closed, and many marchers went on to Trafalgar Square. Some, however, remained; they tore down the railings and entered the park. Loitering and vandalism in the park continued for a few days, sparking revolutionary fears.

5. J. P. Parry, 211. I am indebted for much of my understanding of political personalities of this period to Parry.

6. It is important to remember that there were many different bills over the course of this period, and that an MP who was for one bill might be against another version. I use "pro" or "anti" here for convenience and to contextualize particular excerpts—that is, this speaker is arguing against this reform bill at this particular time. I try also to indicate cases where permanent loyalty to a pro- or

the 1860s (though many Liberals were against reform as well), tended to offer negative threats: the working classes, fit for the franchise but with no hope of receiving it, would lose patriotism and faith in the country. They would emigrate, driving up the price of labor. They would fail to respond to the call of the country in times of distress, refusing to serve as soldiers. The franchise, in these speeches, was explicitly connected to patriotism and national identity. Such reformers began to use the language of citizenship and rights, referring to participation in government as part of "full citizenship." Citizenship, they argued, would engender loyalty and explicitly work against class feeling and class political action—at least on the part of the working classes so admitted. Fitness, then, for at least some of these politicians, implied something like a right on the part of the individual or an obligation on the part of the state.

The move away from a property-ownership qualification in 1832 to that of rental paved the way for the 1860s recognition of the working classes' contribution to the gross national product and also their collective share of income. It was argued that all the funds the working classes had invested in friendly societies, and "their" ability to manage such investment, demonstrated financial competence (a part of fitness) and indicated some stake in the country's well-being that might fitly be recognized with the franchise, analogous to the entitlements of property. Reformers thus made the important move away from linking representation to the payment of the direct cost of government through taxes and toward the more general qualification that every "fit" individual has a legitimate interest in government.

Although secondary to the issue of class representation (and, of course, borough status) in the debates surrounding the first bill, fitness became the primary concern in the second, thus moving substantively closer to twentieth-century notions of citizenship and individual rights. Fitness was morally weighted and broadly defined as the possession of certain abilities. Literacy was important, in order to be able to read and understand materials having to do with the issues, and it was thought that fitness should include some understanding of economics, in terms of both personal money management and the demands of capital and labor, largely as they were understood by the middle classes. "Political economy" as a body of knowledge was largely connected to the capital-labor question, and although knowledge of population management was not explicitly desirable in the individual worker, certainly the goals of political economy were to be evident in the personal practices of

antireform position was particularly marked. It is also important to recall that speeches may be but are not necessarily expressive of a speaker's real beliefs and that often language in a given speech is "party language." Since we are most concerned here with the general logic and recurrent language of these debates, the actual political sentiments of any given member are not particularly important for our considerations.

the laborer and in his domestic economy. Thus, fitness included the ability to sacrifice short-term gratifications for long-term goals, mostly as demonstrated by the rental qualification. Enfranchisement of renters did not simply enlarge the electorate; it also allowed for a greater recognition of upward mobility, particularly among urbanites. Perhaps even more crucially, it connected the demonstration of the citizen's stake in the government with a certain level and type of consumption—that of domestic space. The citizen was in fact to be the Malthusian ideal—a responsible consumer/producer whose desires were shaped by and appropriate to the market.[7] He was not to want too much, and perhaps even more importantly, he was not to want too little (as did, for example, the Irish worker, who was supposedly content with the absolutely minimum food and wages required to sustain life). He was to make decisions based on reason and scientific evidence rather than on emotion. In short, economic fitness focused on two areas of qualification: the ability to manage one's personal finances (an expression of general self-discipline) implied by the rental of an economically eligible property, and the understanding of political economy—a more difficult quality to index.

Indeed, many objected that due to the difference in rental value in various areas, even the first quality was difficult to index. As Mr. Thompson, the liberal MP for Whitby, argued, however, it was the best test available: "those who were selected because of their living in better houses must have possessed the highest qualities as workmen before they could have received the wages which enabled them to inhabit better houses than the majority of their class. They must also have exercised economy . . . and self-denial in not expending their earnings solely on animal enjoyments" (*Hansard's* 157, Apr. 23, 1860: 2227). Moreover, he argued, it was the only test that could be applied practically: "There might be some defects in such a system of selection, but, on the whole, what better mode could be devised? It would be impossible to introduce a competitive examination, or any mode of ascertaining individual merits or qualifications" (ibid.). Proreform MPs also argued in the 1860s that the understanding of larger economic structures connected to the state's weal was demonstrated by working-class involvement in insurance societies. This showed both a collective stake in an economic entity whose well-being was at least nominally related to the well-being of the state and, more importantly, the presence of "self-denial" of the "animal" pleasures among the workers. This would become a key issue, as citizenship was identified with the careful

7. Unlike some earlier works that have focused on biopolitics in the Malthusian terms of sexual desire and reproduction, we are here interested in the larger and more inchoate question of the healthy body's material desires and class tastes, its environment and practices, and their role in citizenship discourse in the period.

management of the body whose needs must never compete with the political priorities of the state.

J. G. A. Pocock argues that modern citizenship constantly attempts to reconcile two views: the elite, Aristotelian view of the citizen as free from materiality, and the view of Gaius, the Roman jurist, that citizens constitute themselves as such primarily through action upon a world of material things. I would argue that these two strands come into particularly sharp and definite conflict in the reform debates and that it is largely out of the Aristotelian ideal that the liberal vision of a split between public and private is constructed. The old ideal of landownership and independent wealth followed a classical, Aristotelian view of citizenship, in which the citizen was to be free of concerns about material or bodily needs. The emerging view of citizenship, however, sought to reconcile a Gaian construction of the citizen through his goods with an Aristotelian ideal that even the economically dependent citizen should show sufficient detachment from his embodied circumstances as to demonstrate control over his immediate wants and desires. Here, self-denial and control over material contingencies substitute for the ideal of wealth sufficient to make such self-denial unnecessary.[8]

Education was early recognized as a necessary (if not sufficient) condition of fitness. In 1831 Whig Prime Minister Charles Grey remarked that "in the nineteenth century . . . the schoolmaster is abroad, and . . . the growing intelligence of all classes is daily receiving new lights" (*Hansard's* 8, Oct. 3, 1831: 943). But literacy, throughout the period, seemed to elites to be a two-edged sword, perhaps leading workers to think revolutionary thoughts. By mid-century, though, the fear of education's propensity to give people ambitions beyond their station had partially given way to a recognition of the power of education and print media as forms of management. Fearful of unionism, elites argued that attention to economic well-being required literacy and some understanding of political economy, and so education (which was soon to become specifically education for citizenship) became a foundation of fitness. In 1866 Gladstone, then Chancellor of the Exchequer, expanded on this theme:

8. Amanda Anderson, in her book on liberalism, cosmopolitanism, and aesthetics, *Powers of Distance,* charts the fascination with and fear of cosmopolitanism that also characterizes the development of the liberal ideal—the citizen should have "detachment," a level of distance and wide experience that allows contemplation of objects, aesthetic or otherwise, from a critical distance, unclouded by personal investment. At the same time, the individual who was too detached, too cosmopolitan in tastes and temper, seemed dangerously rootless and deracinated, without political, national, or personal loyalty or identity. I would argue that this is one way in which the Gaian-Aristotelian conflict plays out—a good citizen is free from the most immediate pressures of immediacy, but not so free as to be unmoored from a recognizable shared materiality deemed crucial to community identity.

> Whether we take education in schools . . . social conduct . . . obedience to the law . . . self-command and power of endurance, shown under difficulty and privation . . . avidity for knowledge and self-improvement—if we apply any of these tests . . . if the working man in some degree was fit to share in political privileges in 1832 he has . . . attained some degree of additional fitness now. (*Hansard's* 182, Mar. 12, 1866: 38)

In short, fitness meant the adoption of upper- or middle-class values, behaviors, and attitudes toward the uses of material and labor. In 1866 Lord Hugh Grosvenor remarked that, in recent years, "which had been marked by such gigantic strides in moral, material, and educational progress, the semi-aristocratic study of politics had become the study of the nation, and the claims of the unenfranchised had been discussed by the unenfranchised themselves in a moderate and intelligent, but in a firm and determined spirit" (ibid., 88).

Fitness and Individuality

The most dramatic change in the debate between 1832 and the 1860s was not the increased emphasis on fitness but the almost wholly new insistence on individuality (and its obverse, anxiety about "massification"). Earlier concerns focused on the lower classes' lack of education and rationality, as well as their vulnerability to bribes—and, of course, fear of revolution. But in the 1860s the ability to act as an individual meant, specifically, the ability (and implicitly, the desire) not to act as one of a class, and rhetoric that demonized the "masses" specifically connected the concept to working-class identity. In other words, it was fear not simply of mass action but of a massed identity or mode of self-construction in which the threat to the state—or even "civilization"—was located. Rioting and other mass demonstrations had long been the focus of the fear of the crowd, but the massified voter sparked a new fear—not of transitory violence to property but of long-term violence to the political mechanism of the state.[9] Significantly, it was his education, financial providence, and access to the press that indicated to liberal reformers that the (especially urban) working man was capable of making reasoned decisions

9. John Plotz's study of the crowd in nineteenth-century literature traces Chartists' early attempts in 1839 to have their demonstrations understood as political discourse in the public sphere. Those who were willing to accept the crowd's actions as such emphasized their reason and nonviolence, whereas those less willing to concede a political voice to the demonstrators emphasized the potential for mass violence. Carlyle's *Chartism,* according to Plotz, constituted the most effective attack on the Chartist demonstrators' ability to have their action taken as political discourse by reclassifying "every apparent speech act of the Chartist crowds . . . as a form of bodily behavior" (138). It is worth noting that Carlyle also defines the crowd as a diseased mass body.

(i.e., based on individual opinion rather than group interests); that is, literacy and some form of property interest qualified the subject as a citizen through his ability to act as an *individual.* And because he was, in fact, an individual, he would not be satisfied with anything less than an individual vote, as opposed to representation through the votes of corporative bodies.

Thus, when worries about working-class preponderance were voiced in the 1860s debates, they were countered with arguments for the individuality of the working man; reformers argued, paradoxically, both that the working classes deserved more representation and that the working man would not vote along class lines. "Individual" was thus defined in opposition to class. Yet an individual must still be contained within the social body and must claim a shared identity, and that identity was to be national. The citizen was indeed to act as an English (or, occasionally, British) subject but was not to vote according to class interests. Individuality, then, is a term with very particular connotations. Although its most obvious connection is with a free-market mindset, its use by most liberal Victorians was quite different. John Stuart Mill, especially, was concerned with fostering citizens who would think and act as individuals, yet he also feared the individual who was too disconnected from society at large. As political theorist Eugenio Biagini puts it, "Both Tocqueville and J. S. Mill feared a democracy of 'monads,' which would lead to a government's undisturbed rule over a mass of isolated individuals. There was the conviction abroad that something more than 'mere numbers' should find representation in parliament, and that between the elector and the representative chamber there should be intermediate forms of collective identity" (23). These forms, he argues, invoke a sense of civic virtue overriding individual needs. Biagini is referring to the debate about representative government, but his remarks are apposite to the definition of individuality as well. Paradoxically, in the presence of a large number of subjects who are *too* individual, they take on the salient characteristics of the "mass" as well: they are unable to act effectively in their own interests and are therefore either too easily governed by a dictatorial state, as Mill feared, or unwilling to govern or be governed for a common good at all. In this second category belonged the pauper or *lumpen*—the numerous folk without any communal loyalties who might combine and act en masse for the most transient of perceived rewards—these were the people who might become the riotous crowd, or mob. Between the individual and the state must indeed be some intermediate form of communitarian identity; lest it be class, reformers urged, let it be citizenship, mediated through the concept of nation.

For most legislators, implicit in fitness was the notion of upward mobility, either already accomplished or with the potential to be, as tending both to inculcate and to demonstrate the values above, and also to diminish (working-) class identification. In short, to act as "an individual" was to act in accordance with the values desirable in an increasingly capitalist state. That the aristocracy should protect its class interests was not seriously and directly challenged until the 1820s, as their interests were considered identical with the interests of England. As English rectitude became identified with the upper middle classes, and as more liquid capital became increasingly significant to the English economy, the right of the large capitalists to act as a class was not significantly challenged in political debate after the 1830s or 1840s, for the same reasons. The broader range of the middle class was so amorphous and varied that it was often considered incapable of class solidarity, as Disraeli remarked. The working class's ability to unionize and combine, however, proved that its members were both fit—in the sense of being able to defer individual interests in favor of long-term and larger goals—and also potentially unfit, because it evoked the threat of large numbers of voters with the proven ability to act in concert against the interests of elites, since by definition the responsible citizen would not undercut those interests, which were seen as identical to the interests of the nation.

Unlike antireformers in 1832, who attacked reform largely on the grounds of balance in representation, those who opposed reform in the 1860s were more likely to attack the fitness of the proposed electorate, granting fitness itself as an acceptable criterion. They argued that the classes under debate were not fit, nor could the granting of rights make them so. Samuel Laing argued, "The object was to admit the intellect of the working classes, as it was found among the artizans and mechanics in the larger towns," but that was the result of setting a higher property qualification, and even that did not work well (*Hansard's* 182, Mar. 12, 1866: 82). A particularly bald statement perhaps best sums up this argument, and I shall therefore reproduce it at some length:

> Mr Lowe:[10] If you want venality, if you want ignorance, if you want drunkenness, and facility for being intimidated; or if, on the other hand, you want impulsive, unreflecting and violent people, where do you look for them in the constituencies? Do you go to the top or to the bottom? . . . it has been said the 10L shopkeepers, and lodging-house keepers, and beerhouse keepers, are an indifferent class of people; but get to the artizan, and there you will see the difference. . . . We know what those persons are who live in small houses . . . and no better law, I think, could have been passed than that which disfranchised them altogether. . . . The effect will manifestly be to add a large

10. Robert Lowe was a hard-line individualist, in many ways a classical liberal, and profoundly antidemocratic. He led the Whig revolt against Gladstone.

> number of persons to our constituencies of the class from which if there is to be anything wrong going on we may naturally expect to find it. . . . The first stage, I have no doubt, will be an increase in corruption, intimidation, and disorder. . . . The second will be that the working men of England, finding themselves in a full majority . . . will awake to a full sense of their power. . . . [They will say] We have our machinery, we have our trades unions; we have our leaders all ready. We have the power of combination. . . . When you have a Parliament appointed, as it will be, by such constituencies so deteriorated . . . I think Parliamentary life would not be worth preserving on those terms. (*Hansard's* 182, Mar. 13, 1866: 147–49)

However, the arguments of the proreform contingent painted a far rosier picture based on the same points:

> William Ewart Gladstone, Chancellor of the Exchequer: Since 1832 every kind of beneficial change has been in operation in favour of the working classes. There never was a period in which religious influences were more active than in the period I now name. . . . The civilizing and training powers of education have for all practical purposes been not so much improved as, I might almost say, brought into existence as far as the mass of the people is concerned. As far as the press, an emancipation and an extension have taken place to which it would be difficult to find a parallel . . . when for the humble sum of a penny, or for even less, newspapers are circulated from day to day by the million rather than by the thousand . . . and carrying home to all classes of our fellow countrymen accounts of public affairs . . . with a sound moral sense, and with a refinement, that have made the penny press of England the worthy companion—I may even say a worthy rival—of those dearer and older papers which have long secured for British journalism a renown perhaps without parallel in the world. By external and material, as well as by higher means, by measures relating to labour, to police and to sanitary arrangements, Parliament has been labouring . . . to raise the level of the working community. . . . Parliament has been striving to make the working classes progressively fitter and fitter for the franchise; and can anything be more unwise, not to say more senseless, than to . . . blindly refuse its legitimate upshot. (*Hansard's* 182, Apr. 12, 1866: 1132–33)

Interestingly, not only education but specifically access to newspapers is frequently mentioned as evidence of literacy, political interests, and a shared culture and values. This culture is national in nature ("the penny press of England") and evokes Benedict Anderson's argument that nationalism depends on a shared printed vernacular and the existence of a cheap and accessible press. In fact, historian Frank O'Gorman notes that in the early nineteenth century, especially by 1830, "The rapidly increasing importance of the printed media and the increasingly sophisticated organization of electoral politics ensured that electors would become increasingly susceptible to issues external to local patrons and external to the constituency. . . . National issues . . . came before 1832 to rival and sometimes even to outweigh the importance of local issues" (292). Electors were already constituting their own identities as voters as part of a larger, national conversation, rather than, as had earlier been true, primarily in terms of local issues and interests.

Although the language of rights and the notion of a fitness qualification are generally mixed together with abandon, one shrewd MP exploited the contradiction. Lord Robert Montagu pointed out that "the most advanced Liberals did not propose to give votes to women, paupers, or children, or lunatics, because they said they were not fit. This was of itself a departure from the ground of natural right, and the laying down of a qualification apart from it—that of fitness." But neither, he argued, were the working classes under discussion fit. The bill, then, "tends to subvert the present distribution of power, and to place it in the hands of the mob—to raise a mere scum to the surface—to enable the poor to tax the rich—the artizans who worked with their hands to place on those who sat still the burden of raising the Revenue—a power which they might not be tempted, perhaps, to use in quiet times, but which in times of excitement would hold out to them an irresistible temptation." He considers the financial qualification inadequate, allowing men of doubtful virtue into the electorate: "As to the character of this new class of voters, in Liverpool a large number of L15 householders were excused the payment of their rates on account of their poverty, and yet 15,068 electors below L10 were now to be added to the constituency." Such "electors" would lack the literacy and the habits necessary to exercise political virtue: "The present constituencies will be subordinated . . . to a majority who are guided by a penny newspaper . . . among whom evil is contagious and self-restraint but little prevails, to whom passion is more seductive than truth and justice" (*Hansard's* 157, Apr. 23, 1860: 2196–97).

Montagu fears the effect of a majority of working-class voters, and here the connection of mass and class is explicit: "No one class should be allowed to rule all other classes. The working classes are generally moderate and reasonable and in possession of wonderful knowledge, considering. . . . But certain Gentlemen had on the other side professed no very exalted opinions of the intelligence of the working classes, particularly on economical questions. They accuse them of believing that the rate of wages depends on the will of the employer" (ibid., 2197). This representation of the pro-union worker as unable to grasp the laws of political economy is a common (and usually negative) one in this period. As workers argued against the laissez-faire insistence that wages must depend entirely on the commodities market, they were accused of lacking the ability to comprehend the "scientific fact" that wages could not be controlled by capital. In turn, whether this was seen as an irrational refusal to address facts or a failure of intellect, this call for higher wages proved their ineligibility for political representation, on the basis of their failure to understand economics.

Montagu ends his discussion by invoking the threat of violence against the very group that seeks reform—a group that he here implies consists of middle-class manufacturing interests: "The employers would perhaps be the first victims marked out for destruction, if once they evoked a spirit and a power which they could neither command nor control" (ibid., 2200). The masses will act as classes, Montagu asserts, and this is not unjust merely because this class will outnumber the others, but because they do act as a mass—either unreasoning or reasoning based on faulty information and a flawed understanding of political economy. Further, he implied, some portion of these masses are actually not a class eligible for citizenship at all but are practically paupers, excused their rates on the plea of poverty. The press here is not representative of a national but a mass-class culture; a penny press is clearly inferior culture, not shared across classes.

It is also significant that this mass class is figured in terms of liability to disease. First, they are a "scum" raised to the surface—evoking imagery of contaminated water described in sanitary campaigns against epidemic disease. Further, this mass seems to be liable to "contagion" of "evil," which is to be aligned with "passion"; their numeric preponderance will create an epidemic constitution of unreason in the body politic as a whole. Lower-class moral quality is often completely aligned with their bodily health in sanitary literature of the day, and this statement builds on that assumption (political commitment is a physicalized "passion"; moral evil is contagious). Many MPs argue that it is precisely the wide dissemination of the penny press (also denounced in this period as "sensational"—again a rhetoric that aligns intellectual with physical experience) that makes it dangerous—too many readers are influenced by a single set of shared (contagious?) opinions (though obviously Gladstone demurs from this position). The language of class warfare is frank, as is the evaluation of possible outcomes. The working class is a physicalized mass—a mass of bodies that "in times of excitement" will override reason. Liberals were as invested in the fear of the mass as Tories or Conservatives, indeed, perhaps more so. And it was the Liberal Party that, riven by fear of mass representation, failed to carry Russell's 1866 bill, leaving the path open for Disraeli's conservative version of 1867 (Parry 214).

Although a few hardy souls boldly asserted the right of the working classes to act in concert, most reformers argued instead that the franchise would discourage class sentiment and, by recognizing the citizen as an individual, encourage him to act thus. Mr. W. E. Forster, the Liberal MP for Bradford, notes, "It is said that the working men as individuals may be loyal, men of sound practical knowledge and good intentions, but that they are to be feared because they are members of large and extensive classes. . . . They are fit as individuals, and not as classes. Why?" And one strategy for stressing the individuality of the working man was to contrast him to the pauper, with whom the opposition consistently attempted to conflate him. There, argued Bradford, lies the real danger to England: "what does this dangerous class consist of? . . . we want to [pacify the Irish and] get rid of pauperism in the country; we want to fight against classes much more to be dreaded than the holders of a L7 franchise—I mean the dangerous classes in our large towns. If we can get into Parliament those who are more immediately above them, we shall be able to legislate more efficiently for them" (*Hansard's* 182, Apr. 16, 1866: 1392–94).

The rhetoric of nation is useful here in creating an "out" group that can be set against the coziness of "our" workers; paupers, criminals, and the Irish, recognized as overlapping classes, are summoned to that end. Most frequently, however, this appeal is carefully buttressed with the assertion that the working classes will not act in concert. Austin Henry Layard continues, "I object altogether to the use of the word 'class' as applied to the working men of this country. Indeed, we generally use the word in a plural, 'classes,' when we speak of them. That is an admission there are as many divisions and subdivisions amongst them as there are amongst any other part of the community." Besides, he notes, "class legislation has been for generations one of the distinctive characteristics" of the Tory opposition (ibid., 1439). In short, class membership is to give way before national identity, within which there is a large, perhaps infinite plurality of individual interests that do not compete with those of the nation. These more local interests are not as threatening as class, either because they are not susceptible to use for identity construction or because those identities are not as readily politicized, or being politicized, do not provide sufficient power with which to mount political action.

Thus, while proreformers were arguing that the working classes both were able to act prudently in concert through Friendly societies and would forgo acting in concert at all, antireformers were forced to concede the working classes' fitness on the very grounds that they claimed proved the working classes did not act like citizens, that is, individually. A good example of this rich confusion, combined with an analysis of the social elements that create, in one MP's mind, a dangerous mass social and political culture, are evident in Mr. Beresford Hope's lengthy attempt both to correct the overgeneralizations of his peers and to construct new and better ways to generalize. He exhorts his proreform colleagues to "deal with him [the working man] as a man, not pat him on the back as a political element, and patronize him. Whatever might be the merits or the demerits of the working man . . . he had one great merit—the honest stand-up, hearty English feeling, detested gammon, and hated to be patronized." He accuses his colleagues of failing to treat workers as human beings and individuals: "They [reformers] were always talking of him and his friends, not as if so many fellow members of society, but as 'the working classes'—namely as a composite something made up of many wants, which had forfeited their individual identity." Hope astutely satirizes the patronizing rhetoric of some reformers, who praised the "working man, as if he were some species of exceptional Darwinian development of human nature. They had patted and patronized him just as if he were a converted African chief at a pious tea party," and he accuses them of not seeing the working man as an individual, "a man with a many sided character, with as many varieties in his natural, moral, physical, social, and financial organization as even the Members of that House."

He then, however, immediately turns to some classificatory rhetoric himself, vowing to describe "who the working man of England really was. He would divide them roughly into three classes"—this being, one supposes, three times better than referring to them as one class. The first class consisted of skilled artisans, to whom, Hope declares, he would be happy to give the suffrage, as "the elite of the working classes." The second class he describes are agricultural laborers, whom he "supposed nobody on either side of the house desired to admit to the franchise." This supposition is based on the lack of mental stimulation supposedly common to country life, "away from all those town influences which tended to form the character of the active as opposed to the passive citizen." Like the rural mobs portrayed in much fiction of the time, including Disraeli's *Sybil,* Eliot's *Felix Holt,* or Kingsley's *Alton Locke,* such workers were thought to be excited by the stimulation of politics to drink, vandalism, and violence, while lacking the ability to make reasoned distinctions based on political values and precepts.[11]

Having dismissed these two large groups out of hand, Hope turns to the third, "a large intermediate class, over whom the battle was really being

11. Karl Marx, writing at about the same time, also decries "the idiocy of rural life" in *Das Kapital.*

fought . . . the large masses of labouring men in towns . . . whose labour was, perhaps, in itself as much mechanical as that of the digger and the delver." These laborers, although like country laborers in their work, were, "by their obtaining higher wages, and from their living under the sharpening influence of towns, within reach of mechanics institutions, and newspapers, of political meetings, and dramatic representations, . . . better posted up." However, he argues, contradicting his earlier statements about workers being too individualized to argue about them productively in the aggregate, "from no fault of their own, they were very much assimilated together. In the upper and middle classes persons could choose . . . their own pursuits, and this produced that healthy and wide diversity of mind which really gave their classes their preponderating influence. . . . But these men, from the very nature of their occupations and circumstances, were more subject to the influence of class feelings" and therefore vulnerable to demagoguery.

Like Adam Smith before him, Hope argues that the nature and conditions of their repetitive labor disallow these workers' political judgments. They work "in continuous grooves and in constant association with their fellow workmen. They . . . must confine themselves to one paper, whether *Reynolds,* an illustrated, or a local journal . . . probably taken in by joint subscription. . . . Their refreshments were obtained in all probability from the same tavern." This aggregation created "class feeling" and therefore, "each single working man was a less unit in the composition of the great national mind and character than each individual of any other portion of the community." He concludes this complex exercise in political algebra by arguing that such workers were utterly ineligible for the franchise, describing them as "the schoolboys of the great commonwealth, who . . . had not, like the typical wise man of Greece, seen the cities of many men and learnt their habits, which formed the true test of a political education" (*Hansard's* 182, Aug. 19, 1866: 1687–89). Notably, though these urban workers have some access to a public sphere, their one tavern and single newspaper forms a public forum too restricted to give them exposure to adequate diversity of opinion. They are a "composite something," a Frankenstein's monster made up of body parts without individual selfhood; these are not the subjects of a liberal state, because they are not subjects at all. Although Hope rejects that definition as adequate for all the laboring classes, it seems to fit perfectly his view of the great majority of the urban workers he describes.

The "active" citizen is urban, shaped by town influences and capable of exercising reason, as opposed to the beast of burden that is the agricultural laborer; on the other hand, Hope falls into the rhetoric he denounces when he calls the urban laborers "very much assimilated together." Further, he believes that their "constant association" and liability to be guided by one (shared) journal means that they cannot be individual selves and so are each a "less unit" in the "national mind and character." He accounts for this inadequacy in terms of development: they are "schoolboys"—minors—who are not ready for the vote. Hope was exceptionally intransigent on reform, an independent conservative (Member for Maidstone) whose driving interest was the Anglican Church as a state institution. He opposed all forms of the Reform Bill and publicly reviled Disraeli for what he saw as a betrayal of principle with the 1867 conservative version of the bill that actually passed (and which avoided enfranchising exactly the classes he identifies as problematic). Still, if he is less moderate in his denunciation of reform, the logic he uses is not significantly different from that of his fellows.

The argument in Hope's speech is perhaps the most explicitly Aristotelian of all these excerpts, befitting his classical liberalism. However, that is a common thread through all these diverse speeches—often manifesting in a confused and somewhat contradictory fashion, it is true, but essentially similar. The mid-Victorian ideal of citizenship, based, understandably, on the aristocratic tradition, insists on the separation of the *res publicae* from the realms of necessity and the body. Thus, the inability of the poorer man to separate himself from his immediate needs—physical, emotional, ultimately economic—disqualifies him from entry into the political or even public sphere. The separation is seen in Cartesian terms—the mind must be cultivated and separated from the body, and this gives the individuality of the bourgeois self. He who is primarily a physical being—a being of necessity—is rooted in the anonymity and universality of the body, its universal physical needs, and thus can only enter the public as an unreasoning and physicalized mass of dangerous flesh, especially when the flesh is corrupt and unhealthy.

Rare indeed was the argument advanced by the Christian Socialist Thomas Hughes, in which he promoted a real class consciousness as appropriate and desirable. As he remarked, Victorians were fond of Samuel Smiles's books in which the self-made man was lauded, and artisans who had "risen to wealth and eminence" by their own efforts deserved respect, but they were not typical. Instead, he praised those who, for him, were more typical workers, whose "principle was to refuse to come out of their class, and to stay and live in it with the view, so far as they could, of lifting the whole bulk of their brethren" (*Hansard's* 182, Apr. 19, 1866: 1706). Despite praising the class-conscious artisan, Christian Socialist writers such as Hughes's friend Kingsley tended to represent such characters as problematic and potentially dangerous, like his character Alton Locke (based on the poet Thomas Cooper), whose Chartist beliefs led him unintentionally to provoke a riot among ignorant rural workers by exhorting them to demand their "rights." Allowing such men direct representation was one way of co-opting such resistance.

Hughes immediately connected class consciousness with moral environmentalism and physical health, relating it to national identity and economic well-being, arguing that "The artizans of this great town were at the present time worse housed than at any period within his memory. . . . The adulteration of the food of the labouring classes had been a great grievance. . . . The people of this country were the worst educated of any free people" (ibid., 1707). However, instead of positioning the working classes as a passive degenerating mass to be medicated, he presents them as consciously assessing their situation and rejecting the state in which they found no stake. The end result, however, is the same as that elaborated by the sanitarians: "Unless Parliament met the people fairly, and gave them a direct share in the representation of the country—made them what were called 'full citizens'—before long we might find the skilled artizans estranged from their country. . . . Their minds would get more and more unsettled; they would continue to leave us [England] more and more" (ibid., 1707–10). Citizenship is here linked to the condition of the body, of its health and physical environment. Bad citizenship produced bad environment, which in turn, willy-nilly, produced bad citizens—sometimes commentators placed the lion's share of blame on the environment and sometimes on the people who inhabited it, but the existence of a direct relationship between the quality of the home environment and citizenship seemed incontrovertible to most commentators in the 1860s. Here the argument is that without representation, these individuals cannot get the physical environment necessary to develop into citizens, and in turn, without that full citizenship, they will fail in patriotism. It is, then, the provenance of the government to provide the sanitary environment that provides the conditions of possibility for citizenship, and this requires public health.[12] Public health was founded on the universal desirability of an essentially middle-class domestic environment. On the other hand, what of those who neither provide nor are nurtured in such a milieu? In the next chapter we will attend both to the central paradigm and to the pathologized outer limits of fitness.

12. Obviously, we must read these excerpts with the awareness that they are suasive rhetorical acts, often incorporating a conscious and disingenuous use of various discursive structures for a purpose. Also, *Hansard's* is not a verbatim record of actual speeches but a reconstruction from notes, which were often modified by members before publication. However, for our purposes, what is significant is the logic behind these arguments and the repeated use of certain tropes and images that clearly reflect a wider discursive formation. Were these arguments voiced by only one or two speakers, they would be interesting, but not useful for this analysis. What I have concentrated on here is samples of widely used and repeated arguments, and I have opted to give long excerpts so as to give the reader something of the discursive setting and rhetorical structure within which such language was habitually used.

2

CITIZENSHIP, CLASS, AND PAUPERISM

> In the largest towns of England, the 10L. men were paupers . . . a mere mockery of a representative body. . . . Was this their conservative body?—the respectable constituency of the parish workhouse? . . . To solicit votes in the lazaretto, or in pauper establishments, was degrading.
>
> —C. Wetherell, MP

> As one of the legislators of the country I am prepared to state that statistics are always false.
>
> —Frank Greystock, character in Trollope's *The Eustace Diamonds*

If the mass was defined by its dangerous contiguity, it was also, as we have seen, loosely defined by elites in terms of class. Yet understandings of class in this period were fairly nascent and often signified quite differently from their meanings in the twentieth century. Here I would like to examine the meanings of class, as the term is being used in these debates. Ultimately, the mass is defined most consistently with the concept of the pauper "class," a group partly defined in economic terms but more saliently by moral and physical characteristics. These characteristics are mediated through emerging ideas of appropriate domesticity; the pauper is without "hearth and home," or the upright behaviors that go with a rooted domestic environment. In short, the definition of class, in relation to citizenship, moves in these debates from being framed at least partly in economic terms to moral ones, then to a matter of domestic practice. The citizen becomes less an economic entity than a member of a certain kind of family in a particular kind of environment.

Mass and Class

In 1832 arguments about fitness related primarily to the artisan and laboring classes—the only classes routinely referred to as such in these debates. But what of that rhetorically and historically privileged group, the middle class, around which the debates of the First Reform Bill largely coalesced? Dror Wahrman has carefully charted the uses of terminologies of the "middle class" during the eighteenth and nineteenth centuries. He points out that the way in which historians have traditionally used "middle class" is deeply suspect, given that there was an "obvious continuity of landed predominance," and he argues that historians have assumed a too-simple relationship between "social being and social consciousness" (5–6). He points out that the "middle classes" are largely a rhetorical construct, historically recent, and with meanings that shifted dramatically over the course of the concept's use. Social reality, he reminds us, does not have a one-to-one—or indeed necessarily any—clear correlation to the representation of that reality (6); the fact that individual Britons represented a powerful middle class and may even have thought of themselves as being part of it has little to do with actual economic conditions. He cites the effects of politics and political language in constructing a "middle-class idiom" that then affects social reality; the "middle-class idiom" is defined as a "rhetoric, which . . . emphasized the singular role of the 'middle class' as the repository of all virtues, the hinge which holds society and the social order together, the major prophylactic mechanism required for a healthy body social and body politic" (46). Wahrman stresses that this rhetoric was "**not** the natural outcome of some pre-formed social and political map, but instead the cumulative aggregate of charged choices made repeatedly by persons sharing certain political values and beliefs" (60, his emphasis).

The languages used as resources by politicians, that is, recirculated by them with particular goals in mind and with particular effects on public language available for constructing a political identity, are themselves shaped in this period by medical discourse, which is itself always already politicized. The lexicon of class, mass, and the working man, as it emerges in these debates, is strongly shaped by the history of uses of the "middle-class idiom" that Wahrman traces with such care; it is also shaped by sanitary rhetoric and that of liberal individualism. The "charged choices" that indeed create the discourses out of which history is made are themselves made from a repertoire that is, in part, already given, out of knowledge systems that are themselves politicized. The irony of elite anxiety about class during the Second (and Third) Reform Bill debates is that elite representations of the "working classes" probably did far more than Chartism to solidify a notion of "working-class interests."

As Wahrman remarks of mobilizations of the language of (the middle) classes in the 1790s, the universal appeal of a language of citizenship "rendered the language of rights fundamentally irreconcilable with the thrust of the 'middle-class idiom,' which, vague though it was, . . . substituted one social group, singled out through some intrinsic qualities, for another" (77). The uneasiness of this relationship between a liberal language of rights and a language of class perhaps explains the uncertainty of "middle class" as a category pertaining to any qualifiers other than beliefs and values that came to be seen as universally desirable over the period. Victorians were generally, for most of the period, quite unable to define a "middle class" in economic terms and tended instead to use terms such as the "middling sorts" or the plural "middle classes" that were used as placeholders for a vague connection between a certain kind of subjectivity, tied to economic status, that was less a class identity in today's sense of the term than simply a concept of the healthy citizen. The construction of a "working class," similarly, came largely from without, and its use oscillated between an economic designation and a pejorative term for those who had not developed the abilities of the citizen; to the extent that "working man" was used positively, it indicated a middle-class subject in an economic position that, almost incidentally, required manual labor.[1]

Class, then, is a term mobilized in complex ways throughout this period, and we are concerned here mostly with elites' definitions used in England. As Patrick Joyce remarks, the language of class is well developed early in the period, but not in its later "primarily 'economic' and conflictual" character (*Visions of the People* 64), and workers, while conscious of class, were not necessarily "class conscious" in the sense that they used class themselves to define an overriding identity. By the time of the 1860s debates, such an understanding is emerging, but in that context, class is often much like gender—an opposition containing a marked term. "Class" by this time is used largely (though not always) negatively in parliamentary debates, and it usually designates the lower classes, who are supposed by the speakers to have exactly the kind of class consciousness that Joyce argues they did not, in fact, yet have. Elites may to some extent have *created* class consciousness, even as they worked to avert it through the construction of citizenship, which, as Marshall later remarked, was not articulated to combat social inequality but to justify it by abating its "less defensible" effects (Marshall and Bottomore 20). Although citizenship and social inequality of classes were not seen to be fundamentally at odds, citizenship and class consciousness were constructed as mutually exclusive. Class consciousness here, then, means lower-class consciousness, defined by

1. Citing Anthony Giddens, Wai-Chee Dimock and Michael Gilmore have analyzed class as a "mediate relation between the economic and noneconomic . . . a set of constitutive relays linking economic identities with social identities. Understood as such, as a relationally derived construct rather than as a self-executing entity, the operations of class necessarily involve an entire spectrum of interdependent terms, whose mutually defining character is progressively obscured as social identities become 'real' . . . to the point where they appear entirely objective and self-evident" ("Introduction" 3). Often the economic elements of class as it is constructed in these debates are almost incidental.

elites to be specifically in opposition to their own interests, which they identified with the nation's interests.

Class as a site of identity construction and potential political mobilization was perhaps most frightening because, unlike other local identities, it was one of the few positions from which it was perceived that a serious opposition might be mounted against nation (just as nation would later become one of the few positions from which to oppose empire). It also seemed to many elites who perceived class as an (inappropriate) mode of subjectivity, rather than in terms of interests, that to recognize working-class status as a potential political position or interest group was to elevate deficiency to the level of an identity in itself. This was class-as-mass, against which elites posed the icon of the individual citizen. But this individual, however iconoclastic in his perception of class and other local identities, was always to identify uncritically with nation, a narrative largely adumbrated by elites.[2]

Thus, although some notion of the upper ranks of society as classed is emerging (or reemerging with a twist), "class" is usually used with a negative instead of a neutral value. As opposed to "the people," or "Englishmen," these lower classes are often identified with amorphous masses of hostile, unreasoning subjects, more animal than human. Although the citizen is an individual, these classes or masses are by definition not composed of individuals; the citizen is a clean and proper component of the social body, but the masses are, precisely, massed bodies, filthy and insufficiently individuated. They are too close—sharing space, water, air, sexual congress. These bodies, being too contiguous, become continuous. The working man is racialized in colonial terms and thus is entangled in the entailments of those terms; hence, the good working man is infantilized and/or feminized, either as a passive someone who needs to be led and managed or as the "schoolboys of the nation" who, with careful guidance and discipline, may be socialized to someday act as adults. Keith McClelland points out that discussions of the working-class demonstrators in the 1860s often revolved around notions of maturity and masculinity, pitting "man-boys" against "proper men" (77). This rhetoric appears in the fiction of the day; in Gaskell's *North and South,* for example, the manufacturer Thornton describes his workers as schoolboys, unable to manage themselves effectively. Either way, even the good working man is a childish creature of emotion rather than reason. The bad working man, on the other hand, is aggressively male, defined by sexuality and violence, more animal than human, incapable of socialization—the Bengali of postmutiny racist literature, the (often Irish) pauper of English urban ethnography.

2. I use the gendered pronoun deliberately, as these debates were held to pertain only to men.

Citizens and Paupers

I would like now to sketch a history of the divisions between those thought to be fit, potentially fit, and unfit for citizenship, and suggest some of the ways in which fitness became tied to a particular domestic environment and individualized body, just as unfitness came to be associated with massed bodies in inadequate domestic spaces. The First Reform Bill debates rather tortuously attempt to distinguish between classes of householders, leaseholders, and respectable and nonrespectable city dwellers, drifting between debates of property versus population as qualifications for a community's representation, and degrees and types of property as qualifications for an individual's right to cast a vote, all in the name of more equitable inclusion within the social and national body. Yet the renegotiation of the national body's individual membership was complicated and restricted by the 1834 Poor Law's creation of a criminalized class of poor, the paupers, who are literally an "out-caste," within but not of the community.

Historian Keith McClelland argues that the notion of the "residuum" defined a "boundary around a particular kind of respectable working-class man"—a domesticated one (98). McClelland contends that this move from property to a more explicit notion of civic virtue based on domestic masculinity resulted in "a narrower political definition of the putative citizen than any dominant strand of popular radicalism had been prepared to draw between 1790 and 1848" (101). (It can be argued, however, that the property qualification, even in 1832, was based implicitly on similar values. Still, the explicit delineation of these values in public discussion may have done much to concretize them in the 1860s.) The bad working man is he who is unsocialized, homeless—literally undomesticated. The social, like the domestic space, is opposed to the economic, public, masculine space, but as its complement and support, producing the conditions that make it viable—and producing, like the good mother, feasible citizens. Class is therefore aligned mostly with negative domestic and gender traits rather than an absolute economic or employment status, although the reform bills would do much to affix a class identity to an economic one.[3]

Membership in the social body, a basis for eligibility for citizenship, had been constructed against the category of the pauper. The pauper was that annoying phenomenon, the outsider within, the indecent poor, or, as Giovanna Procacci put it, "poverty intensified to the level of social danger"

3. Additionally, O'Gorman notes that "there was little to distinguish [in most localities] the occupational structure of radical electors from the occupational structure of the electorate as a whole" (315). Even today, subjective class identity, as measured by self-ascription, is only erratically connected to economic status or occupation (see David Robertson, *Class and the British Electorate*, 80–86).

(158). Although fitness was not yet a basis for enfranchisement in 1832, Britain was beginning the process of revising the concept of the social body to provide for the widespread phenomenon of upward mobility. Class, at this point, was neither clearly articulated nor linked to income; however, respectability was coming to be. Both social-geographical rootedness and financial responsibility were indexed by amount and tenure of rental, and these qualities were in turn supposed to denote education, self-control, and the ability to reason. In turn, respectability, finally endorsed by admittance to the franchise, became something attainable, with effort, for a substantial minority of the population. (Whether this portion of the population cared to attain it is unclear; but it was certainly conceptualized by many elites as a goal desired by this group.)

In the 1830s political reform constituted the subject of national discourse in a new way, suggesting the possibility that any man with the qualification of respectability might constitute himself as a citizen through the exercise of the franchise. Reform constituted the object of that discourse, however, as two divergent groups: one educable, respectable, capable of evolving into a responsible electorate; the other an aggregate of humanity, reduced to a merely physical subjectivity, from whom at best docile obedience to the interests of the electorate and therefore the nation with which they were to identify could be expected. That category was further subdivided into the working poor and the abject pauper mass. Also, in 1832—as the First Reform Bill was being debated and the Poor Law was being researched, the legal category of pauper being formulated—the sanitary movement, spurred by the first cholera epidemic, began.

But how were these paupers to be defined? Edwin Chadwick's amended Poor Law did in 1834 provide a legal definition, but we are concerned here with the hazier criteria of conventional usage that allowed the opprobrium to be more broadly bestowed. In the late 1820s and early 1830s paupers were simultaneously constituted as the "Other" of the citizen and as the site of danger and disease to the social body. When the working classes were constructed as undesirable as citizens, they were paupers. The ultra-Tory Sir C. Wetherell[4] asserted that even the French "did not permit the scale of voters to sink so low [as the ten-pound rule], but they made their voters pass through a kind of filtering stone, the shape of what they called an electoral body, in order to cleanse them from their political filth. . . . By the present Bill, would the citizen mob be made the masters of the citizen Parliament" (*Hansard's* 4, Jul. 6, 1831: 857–58). The ten pounders are not, according to him, the middle

4. Wetherell was one of the most persistent and vocal objectors to any kind of Catholic emancipation or franchise reform. He became so identified in the minds of the voters with the antireform position that his mere appearance in Bristol in 1831 is said to have provoked the famous Bristol riots.

class; "great numbers of these ten-pounders paid their rent weekly—not half-yearly, not quarterly, not monthly—but weekly. Now, here was a class of men, that their landlords would not trust, except from week to week"—so how could they be trusted with the franchise? (ibid., 860). He concludes, "In the largest towns of England, the 101. men were paupers . . . a mere mockery of a representative body . . . was this their conservative body?—the respectable constituency of the parish workhouse? . . . to solicit votes in the lazaretto, or in pauper establishments, was degrading" (ibid., 861). Wetherell's position was deeply felt and his language immoderate—he was famed already as an opponent of the bill and public opinion was against him so he had little to lose; we have to see his sentiments as somewhat exaggerated.

His rhetoric, however, was not wholly atypical. Antireform MP Colonel Connolly, in more moderate but still strong terms, insisted that property and franchise "were, in fact, identical. Those who impeached the validity of the elective franchise, deteriorated property" (*Hansard's* 4, Jul. 12, 1831: 1127). Further, "He knew no better way to decrease the influence of property, than to lower the constituency to the confines of pauperism. One step more would admit all classes to the right of suffrage" (ibid., 1129). These statements may have been intended to be recognized as exaggeration; certainly, pauperism is a highly charged term that is being used at least partly for shock value, but that shock value demonstrates the extent to which pauperism was seen as an essential quality of this portion of the population, rather than a mutable economic property. It also demonstrates the extent to which pauperism was seen as coterminous with epidemic disease, as any pauper establishment becomes comparable to the lazaretto, and vice versa.

Pauperism is a moral category, related to, but not identical with, an economic one. Giovanna Procacci has aptly summarized the stakes in the discussion of pauperism: "Pauperism . . . denotes at once the critical element of the socioeconomic order which economics takes as its end, society's answering riposte to economics, and the line of economic penetration into the evasive substance of the social" (153). She argues that the political significance of poverty in political and economic writings of the mid-nineteenth century stems from the "double meaning" of poverty, "as both the limit to economic discourse and the key to economic conquest" (153). In contrast, at the beginning of the century, pauperism had been seen as an annoying but inevitable by-product of society, a poverty so extreme as to place the subject outside the economy of the community altogether. With the intensification of urban poverty came the need to contain; the insistence on eradicating pauperism altogether, however, arrives with the assimilation of the economic to the political and social body. Paupers remained a social problem in the mid-century precisely because they would not be individuals and good economic subjects—they did not seem to desire the right things or act economically in ways designed to fulfill those desires, and therefore they could not be managed through those desires. Political economy, and all the expert knowledge that mediated between the state and the social, found the limits of their efficacy when confronted with pauperism.

Pauperism was neither just poverty nor just immorality; it was that element of the community that, though produced by society, resisted socialization. Procacci defines pauperism as "the spectre of the mob, a collective, essentially urban phenomenon. It is a composite . . . population which 'encircles' the social order from within. . . . It is insubordinate, hidden from the scrutinizing gaze of any governing instance" (158). In *Aurora Leigh* Elizabeth Barrett Browning describes the poor inhabitants of the city as "The humours of the peccant social wound. . . . They clogged the streets, they oozed . . . in a dark slow stream, like blood" (134–35), using both disease and fluid imagery to illustrate the idea of a dangerous mass. (I will consider this fluid imagery more extensively in a later chapter, with reference especially to Dickens.) Procacci notes that pauperism as a concept is not essentially economic: "rather than a certain level of poverty, images of pauperism put the stress principally on feelings of fluidity and indefiniteness" (158). This sense of a mobile, mutable force that is everywhere and nowhere is actually quite unfounded. Although Henry Mayhew's casual laborers in the classic Victorian ethnography *London Labour and London Poor* (published first in 1849–50 in article form in the *Morning Chronicle* and in 1851 as a book) are "nomadic," restlessly wandering through the city, careful attention to his text demonstrates that these nomads follow a predictable pattern and tend to move constantly within rather small territories. But the apparent lack of rootedness, of investment in a particular domestic and geographic location, placed these people beyond the pale of socialization.

Thus, to the extent that the working classes could be conceived as citizens, they were not paupers, and vice versa. Marx, champion of the proletariat, makes clear distinction between the working classes and paupers, or *lumpenproletariat,* "a mass sharply distinct from the industrial proletariat, a recruiting place of thieves and criminals of all sorts, living upon the offal of society, people without a definite mode of making a living, *gens sans feu et sans aveu*" (*Class Struggles* 58). For Marx, *lumpen* are inexcusable (though he also expresses an ambivalent admiration for them) precisely because they are incapable of class feeling, having allowed themselves to be set against the proletarian revolutionaries in 1848. But what makes *lumpen* unavailable to communitarian class identification is precisely the same lack of socialization that made them incapable, as British elites thought, of citizenship. Without property, their loyalty can be suborned; they have nothing to protect. Too much a mass, too easily led, they are also too disconnected from larger economic structures to be reliable. Without a definite mode of making a living, they are also without hearth and home, undomesticated, unsocialized. Like Dickens's poor boy Jo in *Bleak House,* they are constantly "moving on." In these moments, Marx shows himself rooted in the same ways of thinking about citizenship as his liberal contemporaries, for whom the home and family (and by implication, private property) are the preconditions for socialization. They are independent—not to be confused with individuality in the sense involving Mill's ideal of independence of opinion. Independence here is precisely the type of individuality that is not wanted—independence from social control because economic needs and desires considered appropriate to the citizen have not been internalized. And even when the pauper is economically dependent, on charity, for example, that dependence is believed to create no responsive socialization, as it does in those who depend on an employer's or a community's approval for their livelihood. We are returned to Biagini and the observation that individuals with no communitarian identities become masses as well.

Domesticity and the Citizen

The importance of the home in this rhetoric cannot be overestimated. The realm of the body, of reproduction, of necessity, beginning with Malthus's emphasis on population and becoming acute with the advent of epidemic disease, becomes an urgent public issue, an unavoidable political problem. This problem represents the intrusion of the private and domestic into the public sphere that engaged the anxiety of those steeped in the Aristotelian tradition of statecraft. The home is the fostering ground of common values. But despite the importance of the home, the material realm, public identity depends on a careful separation of the private from the public, which the existence of property supposedly guarantees its owner—that is, sufficient freedom to weigh in disinterestedly on matters of public importance. At all costs, these bodily issues must be driven back into the domestic sphere where they belong, and in which such disorder should be contained and disciplined. But before this could take place, these troublesome subjects would have to have domestic privacy in the first place.

Paradoxically, by the late 1850s, it was quite clear to most liberals that the only way to accomplish that goal was to organize a widespread and coherent intrusion into the private domain of the poor, in order to teach them how to keep their private affairs—whether the state of their drains or the state of their bodies—where they belonged. Put another way, the realm of necessity, which had always been a crucial but invisible, mystified, and disavowed part of politics, was surfacing with a vengeance as capitalism and liberalism brought economics, politics, and the expanding polis closer together—hence, the sudden insistence on an absolute separation of public and private, the enforcement of newly strict gender divisions, and the solidification of a depoliticized and feminized realm between public and private—the social—which would focus on the inculcation of proper domestic habits among the poor, from which, it was reasoned, civic virtue must follow.[5]

By the late eighteenth century "the association of women with both domesticity and virtue was fast becoming a cultural commonplace" (Poovey, "Social Constitution" 47). As private bodies defined by reproductive capacity who were not compensated economically for their labor, middle-class women were definitively in the realm of nature. But we would also do well to remember that there is no necessary connection between the middle classes as such and domesticity—that this connection was created in relation to other narratives about class and specific historical and political contingencies. Dror Wahrman points out that before the 1830s the middle classes were more likely to be identified with the masculine realm of business than a feminized domesticity (381–82). However, in novelistic writing, a domestic middle class was more commonly represented. After 1832 these genres began to merge in their construction of the middle classes, and by the 1840s it was firmly instantiated

5. Nor is this view of the social unique to the eighteenth and nineteenth centuries. Indeed, we are the heirs to this set of unspoken contradictions. Hanna Fenichel Pitkin points out that the philosopher Hannah Arendt, though one of the most voluble theorists on the subject of "society," "the social sphere," and "the social"—terms that sometimes overlap and are sometimes differentiated in her work—provides us with no clear definition of the social. What does emerge in Pitkin's careful reading of Arendt's work is the following: the social is oppressive, feminized, infantilizing. It inculcates conformity and may contribute to the phenomenon of mass man or mass society. It arises out of the (for Arendt, inappropriate) irruption of private, domestic concerns—concerns rooted in the body—into the political sphere and, by turns, an inappropriate intrusion of public into private concerns. It is also—though again, Arendt is not very clear on this—related to the development of a large market economy that promotes conformity and personal irresponsibility in the face of what are seen as impersonal and pervasive market forces. These two strands, for Pitkin, are never clearly linked. Arendt's concept of the social is clearly related to the concept that I am discussing here. What perhaps blocks Arendt's inclination to delineate its nature more fully is her insistence on the rigid separation of the domestic, material world of necessity and the abstract, moral world of political action—an action she sees as being dependent on a preexisting self that is separate from the social. Habermas indulges in this same Aristotelian concept of citizenship, and it is my contention (and certainly not mine alone) that this concept is elitist and fundamentally antidemocratic in its persistent mystification of the inextricable ties of the material to the political and the inseparability of public and private sphere. Arendt is quite right when she recognizes—though with the same fear that led Victorians to believe in the autonomy of the social, the public, and the private—that the social emerges from "the rise of the 'household' (*oika*) or of economic activities to the public realm" (in Pitkin 11). She calls it an "'unbearable perversion of the human heart' because it invades 'an innermost region in man which until then needed no special protection.' . . . The social is, then, 'neither public nor private' but some kind of 'curiously hybrid realm'" (ibid., 15).

(Wahrman 406–8). Just as middle-class virtue was aligned with the domestic woman, class itself was created as an identity rooted in the home.

Indeed, the habitus of class identity is formed within the family, but that identity is lived only in comparison with other identities in a larger social group—one is interpellated as lower-class when one interacts with a person of a class above one. It is the triumph of a bourgeois self-construction adumbrated in the literary domain that it becomes, in a very short time, the epistemological basis of class politics. By the time we come to the 1860s debates, domestic values are so much the mark of middle-class-ness—which is less a discrete category than the very definition of virtuous citizenship—that citizenship itself is identified with domestic femininity, as is English national character. The middle classes become an honorary category related to the possession of a certain character, a potentially universal nonclass as opposed to the "classes below."

These domestic qualities were necessary for the development of private man. But like the world of material necessity, they—and the women responsible for them—were to be cordoned off in the private sphere. Put another way, like the women and slaves whose labor in the domestic arena made possible the ideal Greek citizen's freedom both to claim a place in the political domain and to devote his energy to the consideration of the responsibilities of that place, women and laborers in Victorian Britain presented a problem if they claimed separate representation. Women's biological difference presented a way to classify them as bound to that private world of biological necessity, as they had been for Aristotle's culture. The private sphere was maternal to the nascent male citizen. As the growing popularity of "public schooling" for the middle-class male of this period attests, the emergence into masculinity was connected to the splitting of the male subject into two identities: the domestic subject or "family man," whose moral virtues were shaped by a maternal ethics of sympathy and care, and a civil and economic subject, whose identity was homosocially determined and whose virtues were "masculine" ones. Some of these virtues included a militaristic ability to lead and follow, loyalty to class, school, and nation, competitive values, and increasingly, with the influence of Muscular Christianity, an athletic body that was sufficiently reliable so as to free the subject from the necessity of reflecting upon its needs.

In other words, the male child was expected to cultivate two subjectivities—public and domestic—that were sustained and shaped by quite different values. Yet the public self was formed on the basis of the domestic self, whose values were seen as foundational, human values. The lower-class man, however, either had to be made able to create and maintain his own division between public and private, or a reason had to be found that explained his inability to do so. It was, perhaps, natural, then, that both such a reason and its remedy would be sought in the domain of physiology (and often blamed also on the inadequacies of working-class women's maternal and domestic abilities). The social technology of public health set as its task the reclamation of the pauper mass, socializing and individualizing the masses so that they might be reintroduced into the domain of the economic (and from there, the political).

The anticitizen was a wanderer, without home attachments, and therefore without potential for citizenship. Over the course of the century, such vagabondage is biologized and, later, racialized. The biological degeneration is environmentally rather than purely genetically determined; since it comes from outside the organism, even though it may then become hereditary, it is meliorable. The unregenerate mass, like the unregenerate environment, must be penetrated by the scientific gaze, which takes up information as statistics and returns it in the form of education, housing reform, and medical intervention. Against the fit body of the individual citizen is set the massing of (dirty, diseased) working-class bodies; against a politics and economics of individualism is set the specter of class action. And somewhere in between are those who are newly social citizens becoming ready (but not yet) to be political citizens; in short, this discourse is avowedly as much about the function of a social citizenship involved in becoming part of civil society as it is about the franchise. In the next chapter, we will see how this discourse of mass and class developed, in relation to public health, and how public health became a means of addressing this problematic population.

3

DISEASE, THE SOCIAL BODY, AND FITNESS

> Unhealthy localities attract certain classes of people, and overcrowding renders cleanliness and ventilation very difficult, even if the people were disposed to put them into operation. Unhealthy houses act upon the people, and the people re-act upon the houses, and thus cause and effect are interchanged, and the result is disease mortality, demoralization and crime.
>
> —"Sanitary Condition of the Epidemic Districts in the United Parishes of St. Giles and St. George"

> The Cholera comes—Rejoice! Rejoice!
> He shall be lord of the swarming town!
> And mow them down, and mow them down!
>
> —Charles Mackay

As the citizen came to be defined against the pauper, and by a particular kind of domestic practice, the pauper was coming to be defined chiefly in terms of a threat to the physical as well as moral health of the social body. The rhetoric of sanitary reform and of franchise reform dovetail early on in the 1830s formulation of the fitness problem, and the morally desirable practices of domesticity that are urged on the pauper are sanctioned by the mandates of public health. Just as the massed public opinion of the unfit is thought to endanger the body politic and social, the massed physical bodies of paupers in overcrowded slums are seen as matrices of epidemic disease, and their domestic circumstances as a threat to the moral and physical welfare of the nation. As the franchise is increasingly debated in terms of its potential tonic effects on the unfit, fitness itself comes to be insistently physicalized, and the management of the social body is elaborated through the bureaucratic machinery of public health.

Cholera and Reform

Some of the associations between health and citizenship can be traced to the aleatory historical connection between reform and disease. At the same time as the First Reform Bill debates heated up in the summer of 1832, a new threat arrived. The first world pandemic of cholera reached the shores of Britain in 1831 and London in 1832; it competed with the reform bill for the front pages of the newspapers. The public was quick to make the connection between cholera and reform. Cholera had been immediately associated with poverty and immorality as a result of existing medical and political beliefs; it was also quite publicly connected with reform, in part simply because of timing and in part because of rhetorical strategies initiated by the Church of England and reflected in response by labor radicals, such as Henry Hetherington, editor of *The Poor Man's Guardian.* The Church declared that "national sin" had caused cholera and declared a day of fasting, whereas labor radicals suggested that it was resistance to reform and abuse of the working people that had brought the epidemic down upon Britain. (Hetherington, among others, pointed out that fasting was not an unusual activity for laborers under ordinary conditions, and he suggested that those classes should observe a day of feasting instead.) Meanwhile, the public health movement, then led by sanitarians such as Edwin Chadwick (who had no medical training), pointed to the filthiness of the poor as the cause of disease, rather than the starvation the radicals claimed, or the divine wrath identified by conservative Churchmen.[1] Parliamentary speeches, sermons both preached and printed, and letters to the various editors trumpeted the connection between cholera, public health, and parliamentary reform.

Whereas the poor and working-class radicals reacted against both sanitarians and clergy in 1832, lumping their interests together, radicals of both middle- and working-class origin later in the century tended to support the public health movement, seeing common ground in the desire to fight disease and provide a better environment for the poor. Public health became key in what came to be called the Condition of England question, in the struggle of the lower classes for inclusion in the national body, indeed, in the very definition and identification of nation with a middle-class, cleanly, British body, which, in the late 1850s, would become racialized as specifically English. For the remainder of the period, charitable, housing, and labor reform would focus on health, above all other issues, including crime, as that which bound the "two nations" into a single body through a communicative medium of disease.

1. For more on the relation between medical and clerical discourse surrounding the cholera epidemics, see Gilbert, "'A Sinful and Suffering Nation.'"

As the narrative of shared national identity organizes itself around the notion of citizenship versus class, so does the concept of a radically connected social body, in which all of the constituent parts have the ability to affect one another—or, conversely, have no ability *not* to. Disease highlighted the vulnerability of bodies placed in contiguity by urban congestion, or by capitalism—cholera carried off both paupers and respectable victims, and Muscular Christian minister and sanitarian Charles Kingsley, for example, in "Cheap Clothes and Nasty" wrote of starving tailors contaminating the clothing of the upper classes with their diseases.[2] This continuous, mass body was necessarily grotesque—defined by its excretions and lower bodily structures.[3] Closing the body's inappropriate openness, managing its excretions, controlling its desires—these have long been part of the socialization process in modern societies.[4] In the nineteenth century these socially determined processes, which had historically developed in part as class signifiers, came to be seen as universally desirable and intimately related to statecraft. What had been the insensibly absorbed habitus of the bourgeoisie would become a formalized curriculum—a set of precepts about morality and hygiene—taught by professionals to the formerly unfit.

Public health arose as a technology for managing the health of this social body. As modernity highlighted a physical connection between classes, the emergence of what would become mass culture—the penny newspapers, cheap clothes and nasty, and so on—also created a shared consumer culture wherein social differences were marked more and more subtly. This gave rise both to anxiety about reinforcing boundaries between classes and to efforts

2. As Peter Stallybrass and Allon White observe, "The police and soap . . . were the antithesis of the crime and disease which supposedly lurked in the slums." But that policing is effected through the bourgeois gaze, which is then implicated in its object: "Thus, even as a separation of the suburb from the slum established certain class differences, the development of the city simultaneously threatened the clarity of that segregation . . . and the fear of that promiscuity was encoded above all in terms of the fear of being touched. 'Contagion' and 'contamination' became the tropes through which city life was apprehended" (134–35).

3. Mikhail Bakhtin has defined the grotesque body celebrated in carnival as a body defined in terms of its openings and its "lower strata": digestive, excretory, genital, and reproductive. In other words, it is a body defined by its liminal structures and states in which inside and outside merge. In carnival, this liminal aspect of the grotesque body is presented directly to view, challenging ideologies that privilege orderliness and authority/ownership, with their doxa of the closed and impenetrable body dominated by reason and will. In the Victorian era two kinds of bodies definable as grotesque were the diseased body and the body of the prostitute—often one and the same. Both were defined chiefly by their permeability, and both became the objects of the gaze. However, they did not do so only in the context of carnival, but in the context of policing and the reinforcement of the boundaries they threaten; in lock hospitals, *cordons sanitaires,* blue books, and clinics, the grotesque body was segregated from society, measured and weighed, sometimes destroyed.

4. See Norbert Elias's *The Civilizing Process* for a detailed study of increasing bodily and emotional self-control and the removal of bodily processes involving secretion, sexuality, or the digestive process from public view over the entire modern period.

to eradicate those boundaries, bringing all within a unified civic culture that would protect social hierarchy without inspiring class sentiment. This delicate art—that of bringing workers within the social body while retaining social and economic inequality—is the art of civil society under capitalism. And citizenship begins with technologies of the self—creating a unifying habitus of the body, which in turn creates and reinforces bourgeois tastes in consumption. If nationhood is a rhetoric, citizenship is a set of social and cultural practices that connect that rhetoric to the economic and political.

Reform as Political Sanitation

As we have seen, MPs were initially concerned about fitness conferring eligibility for citizenship. But in a chicken-and-egg argument, some believed that fitness could also be produced by citizenship. Citizenship itself was then, by many reformers, envisioned as a mode of management, a political sanitizing of the social body. These individuals contended that participating in government would facilitate the new citizens' internalization of the system of government as a means of self-regulation or self-government. Thus, the citizen self-regulates in a manner that advances the interests of the state, which in turn is expected to advance the interests of the citizen. Typical of this argument was the implication that masses of workers concentrated in urban space were a source of danger unless they became "governmentalized." As Whig-Liberal Edward L. Bulwer put it in 1831, "in large towns, the more persons were excluded from voting, the more enemies the Constitution had. Those who were not electors, were a disorderly and disaffected rabble; all those who were raised to the rank of electors were converted into citizens, and interested in the preservation of the public safety." On the basis of this theory, he argued for the most extensive franchise compatible with setting at least a minimal qualification:

> There was no better collateral means to preserve good order, than . . . to encourage those who had none [votes], to exert industry and energy to attain them. It was consequently wise, to allow the qualification to be so fixed, as would enable the poorest man, by the exercise of these qualities, to elevate himself to the consideration of a citizen, from that of being one of a disorderly mob." (*Hansard's* 6, Aug. 25, 1831: 609)

Here, although the citizen is still expected to attain a minimal level of fitness, it is implied that citizenship itself creates fitness, rather than the other way around. However, in both debates, references to Frankenstein's monster were used by antireformers to deride the attempt to ennoble a dangerous aggregate of corrupt parts, an aggregate with power but without fitness to exercise it. Tory leader Sir Robert Peel said in 1831 that reformers "had created a power, endowed, like the Monster in the novel, with tremendous physical energies, and when they found that they could not subject those energies to the control of moderation and reason—then it was that they shrunk appalled from their own success" (ibid., 636–37). The effect of letting loose such a monster was nothing less than the erosion of the body politic's humanity itself, dragging the state down to a bestial and monstrous level: "The introduction of that class into the constituency would deprive property and intelligence of their due influence. . . . It would have the effect of degrading the Representation" (ibid., 637). Further, it was argued that not only would the franchise fail to confer the qualities appropriate to its exercise but its extension would also eliminate the motivation to develop such qualities. Moderate and well-respected Irish Conservative James Whiteside was still arguing this position in 1866: "It has been said we must elevate the working classes by giving them the franchise. No such thing. . . . They may elevate themselves by their economy and their prudence, and if they can do so and get the franchise, then it is a wise and politic arrangement." At this point, however, the image of the "bestial" elector intrudes again: "I cannot, however, understand the principle which says that we are to go lower and lower in the scale of civilization to the electors instead of offering them an inducement, by prudence and proper conduct, to elevate themselves" (*Hansard's* 182, Mar. 13, 1866: 199). The franchise was a tonic that could produce political health, whether as reward or as prophylaxis.

Others argued that the good effects of citizenship could be had with balanced representation, without losing elite control by numerically increasing the electorate. In 1831 Dudley Rider, the Tory Earl of Harrowby, was frank about the advantages of such a system: "I rejoice that popular franchise has formed a part of the constituency of this country . . . because it has tended to give the people that exalted idea of their own freedom which distinguishes them from the nations of other countries, because it has given them an interest in the affairs of State, and fostered, in all classes, even the most humble, a spirit of pure patriotism." Still, he worried about the effects of this "exalted idea" on the excitable masses: "with a constituency universally popular . . . Whenever any popular excitement takes place at the time of a general election, will not nearly the whole House represent only the temporary opinion and passions of a majority[?] . . . what will become of stability, the great element of social and political happiness?" (*Hansard's* 7, Oct. 4, 1831: 1163–64). Patriotism is a desirable excitement, manageable to useful ends, but an excited and empowered mass would be dangerously unstable.

Others, however, while granting there is no right to the franchise, uphold reform on that very principle of management. This argument only becomes stronger as the century wears on, and by the 1860s it is perhaps the strongest pragmatic argument. James Graham remarks that "inequality of condition is one of the necessary and inevitable accidents of society" and that therefore he has never believed that there is a universal right of suffrage. Still, he argues, given the "growth of education and intelligence," it is correct to extend the franchise, as "The advantages to those thus admitted consists in the increased self-respect, the diminished class feeling, the closer contact with higher cultivation, the lessened temptation to illegitimate self-assertion" (*Hansard's* 182, Apr. 16, 1866: 1665–66). So both sides agree that it is desirable to manage the working classes, not simply to control them but to make them better citizens, that is, better self-managers.

Conversely, the effects of continued disenfranchisement are presented not as stasis but as degeneration. The MP, liberal littérateur (and member of the Apostles) Monckton Milnes[5] argued that artisans would have no motivation for educating themselves if they were not to be able to "participate in the political duties and privileges incident to its [their country's] Constitution. They would either separate their political from their intellectual life, or in proportion as their intellectual life was developed they would become discontented at being excluded from the political machine to which they belonged." In contrast to antireformists' arguments that workers' empowerment was potentially perilous, he argues the opposite: "The spectacle of any large class of society separating themselves from the political action of that society was always fraught with danger, especially when that was an educated, literary, and accomplished class, whose influence ought, if properly directed, to improve the political condition of their countrymen" (*Hansard's* 157, Apr. 23, 1860: 2218–19).

Sanitation as Political Therapy

We have said that liberal governmentality requires the ability of the state to know what its subjects are doing and to manage them in order to eliminate undesirable and encourage desirable behaviors. By the 1860s, medicine, along with its subfield, vital statistics, was one of the most highly privileged of the systems of expertise that made this model of government possible. Whereas in 1831 MPs' speeches identified the elimination of violent mob activity as a primary goal and the promotion of economically desirable activity as a secondary goal of this management, speeches in the 1860s implied a much more complex and clearly defined set of goals for working-class behavior, as well as

5. Milnes continued to support the franchise throughout his career, including during his tenure in the House of Lords, as Baron Houghton.

the elimination, rather than simple control, of pauperism. Many of these goals are explicitly to be reached through sanitary strategies (such as better housing, cleanliness, and the elimination of food adulteration), and these, in turn, are openly related to the franchise. Statistical data is invoked frequently to both define problems and support solutions, as is personal observation.

Medical knowledge is not simply used as support for arguments about government but as a mode of government itself. Members' speeches frequently refer to personal contact with medical observers to legitimate points they are making and often metaphorically identify the statesman with the medical observer. In this way they claim both the credibility of empirical knowledge and the privileged gaze of the medical man. Robert Lowe observed that "It is the duty of the Government, like any other physicians, to study the case. . . . Otherwise they are acting like a physician who spends his time in mixing drugs and sharpening lancets and never takes the time to see what is the matter with his patient" (*Hansard's* 182, Mar. 13, 1866: 155). And Sir William Hutt (free trade advocate, MP for Gateshead) claimed that he "went among the coal-whippers at their labour, and entered the gin shops; . . . he visited them in their own homes, and he saw also the medical men who were in the habit of attending them . . . and he supported the Bill" (*Hansard's* 182, Apr. 16, 1866: 1683). Doctors and surgeons began to emerge as important characters in novels portraying political struggles in the mid-century: Harriet Martineau's novel *Deerbrook* features a doctor who disagrees with his patron on sanitary issues and forfeits both his fees and his peace, as he becomes a target of violence by uneducated laborers; he is vindicated when fever breaks out among the poor who have failed to follow his advice. (He is a precursor to Eliot's Lydgate, in *Middlemarch,* who does not stand quite as firm in his conflict with his political patron.) *Bleak House* finally marries off Esther, its exemplary domestic woman, to a rising young doctor whose practice is also among the poor. Doctors in this period come to take a role alongside the minister as social heroes in the novel.

The position of the medical profession—and this period is one in which professionalization is the decisive characteristic of medical practice—had been revolutionized over the three decades intervening between the first and fourth cholera epidemics. This was partially because of the energetic efforts of professional bodies but was also in large part due to the profession's claiming of a distinct space and part in the creation of the social. Whereas medics had been largely silent in the first epidemic, by the second epidemic of 1848 they were vocal not only about the causes of disease but also about their unique ability to diagnose the needs of the public.[6] Part of their claim was based on

6. I use the term "medics," following Frank Mort's example, to designate all of those engaged in medical practices and perceived to be legitimate medical practitioners by the general public in this

the connection between physical health and morality; since moral health required physical health, increasingly seen as the purview of medical experts, medics were in a unique position to speak to and improve the moral fitness of the body social. Edmund Parkes, author of *Practical Hygiene,* which medical historian Mark Harrison describes as "the standard text for military medical men in Britain and the colonies in the 1860s, 70s and 80s" (52), has this to say about the role of the public health official: "For a perfect system of hygiene we must combine the knowledge of the physician, the schoolmaster and the priest, and must train the body, the intellect and the moral soul in a perfect and balanced order" (ibid., 53).

Epidemics, especially cholera, were both a help and a hindrance to medics in achieving this empowerment in the public domain. On the one hand, they focused public attention and generated sufficient alarm to push for sanitary measures and to build, over thirty-four years, a board of health with some legal powers. Epidemics gave medics a platform to speak about public policy issues, rather than just the private issues of individual health that had traditionally been their domain. However, since epidemic disease was so strongly associated with abject poverty, it was difficult to separate the health laws from the administrative machinery of the Guardians of the Poor. This meant both that public health was considered an underclass issue, rather than one for the general public, and that means of enforcement of public health initiatives were initially extremely limited. It required the discourse of moral environmentalism and its implications for political fitness and racial degeneration of the working classes, combined with the more specific threat of cholera as "trigger," to push through legislation granting more power to the board and urging attention to food adulteration and housing reform, and it took more than three decades to do it. (Although there was a significant health act in 1848, also spurred by the threat of cholera, Parliament failed to give the board "teeth" until the act of 1866—during a cholera epidemic.) The pathologizing of the pauper and concomitant focus on the citizen's body enabled medics to make the connection between their knowledge of disease and the political health of the nation. Working class readers were told,

> [Cholera] is checked by [man's] skill and his firmness. . . . It will finally be banished from the well-governed regions of the earth altogether. First, it will disappear from those which it has most recently attacked [i.e., England];—and, in the end, as the blessings of civilization extend themselves to every region on which the rain from heaven falls, or the sun of heaven shines; and as man improves in knowledge, virtue and power, and by degrees converts vast spaces

period. This would include not only physicians (doctors) but also surgeons, apothecary-surgeons, and apothecaries.

> now neglected into spots of fertility and happiness, and is himself raised in the scale of creation,—not the cholera only, but all the most severe febrile diseases, will probably be utterly banished from this globe. (SDUK 202–3)

The moral onus of disease was shifted in this sanitary rhetoric from the person to the place in which he or she lived, which had the desirable effect of spreading responsibility for disease to a larger community. However, it also reinforced a sense of environmental determinism that figured the people who lived in such places as a passive aggregate with limited agency, subjectivity, or morality. The discourse of moral environmentalism thus conflated unhealthful living conditions with the moral and physical degradation of the population to the level of a mass. Although this confirmed the vision of the poor as incapable of exercising citizenship, it also implied a remedy that might bring such creatures within the pale of those who could develop into citizens over time. Moral environmentalism contributed to the conception of healthful environment as a prerequisite of citizenship; health, like literacy, came to be understood as something the developing person must have access to as a necessary precondition for cultivating the qualities required for citizenship, including individuality.

The Dangerous Body: Crowding and Pauperism

In the 1830s sanitarians had focused on cleanliness, leading to acknowledgment of the need for sewerage and adequate supplies of water. Over the next two decades the problems of sewer engineering focused increased attention on geographic features, while the housing movement simultaneously focused on the landscape of the structure and interior of the built environment. Thus, from a focus on individual bodies and their interiors, sanitary studies moved to places—with which their inhabitants were identified. The bodies of the poor were superimposed on the environment.[7] As the city itself came to be described as a body, with organs of circulation and elimination, the poor came to be identified with inappropriately eliminated excreta. The bodies of the poor were messy, embarrassing bodies, aligned with what Mikhail Bakhtin defined as the grotesque and Julia Kristeva as the abject—defined by their openings and inappropriate exposures and excretions. They were also a mass body, joined through those openings and excretions in dangerous and repulsive ways. Mid-century sanitary discourse cited not only the pathogenic properties of such massed bodies but also their moral degeneracy.

7. For a detailed discussion of the spatialization of epidemic disease, especially cholera, in the nineteenth century, see Gilbert, *Mapping the Victorian Social Body*.

Violence, alcoholism, incest, unwed pregnancy, prostitution, and property crime were thought to be a few of the most common behavioral "products" of this massing, as cholera, typhus, and other fevers were their epidemiological products. Both were social problems because their effects could not be contained and affected the larger social body. Dr. John Sutherland, who worked under Edwin Chadwick, quotes the Statistical Society on overcrowding: "'all ages and both sexes, fathers and daughters, mothers and sons, grown up brothers and sisters, stranger adult males and females, and swarms of children, the sick, the dying and the dead, are herded together with a proximity which brutes would resist'" (in Sutherland 7). Such inadequate policing of the body's boundaries led to addiction, violence, and disease (which, in turn, were thematically related to social and political irresponsibility, as we shall see in later chapters discussing Gaskell, Eliot, and Dickens).

By the 1860s the two most important factors in a healthy environment were considered to be the allocation of a certain amount of physical space to each individual, that is, physical separation, and the related absence of wastes. The necessity of space was indicated both by the need of the body to continually excrete its waste products, through respiration and perspiration as well as urination and defecation, and also by the moral requirement of privacy. Chadwick and Southwood Smith, in their capacity as official spokespersons for public health, estimated that "health and strength cannot be maintained in a breathing space of less than from 700 to 800 cubic feet"—a typical observation (247). Only in such an environment could a person properly breathe—or develop the sense of individuality required for citizenship. The emphasis on respiration and the continuous excretion of impalpable wastes highlights the ever-present dangerousness of the body itself—a significant difference from the earlier focus on nuisances such as dung heaps, wherein it was specifically urine and fecal waste, both visible and palpable, that were dangerous and not the bodies themselves.

Chadwick and Smith exhort the public to open their windows: "A neglect of ventilation leads to such a noxious atmospheric deterioration when any considerable number of persons are collected together. It is well known, in a general way, that this is caused by the exhalations or the secretions of the animal body, and essentially by those of the lungs and skin."[8] In addition to the feared "carbonic acid gas" that living things exhaled, "there is a highly nox-

8. Disease was widely thought in this period to be caused by decaying substances in the air. This "miasmatic theory" was key in mobilizing the removal of dung heaps and other nuisances. Here we see a new emphasis on the body itself as a continuous producer of decay. (Germ theory, the theory of a specific causal agent of disease, would not emerge until the 1890s, though medics such as John Snow and William Budd had argued as early as the late 1840s that diseases could be caused by specific agents, perhaps fungal in nature.)

ious [substance], which, if it be collected by the condensation of the expired vapours [of the breath], and kept for a few days, becomes decomposed, and emits a strong putrid odour; and so again in the case of the skin, there is, without a moment's cessation, emitted a vapour . . . which, like the vapour from the lungs, contains effete, that is, decayed, animal matter." As they point out, the very design of the human body points to the dangers associated with its excretions: "That these animal substances are most noxious to the living body, will be immediately inferred from the fact, that one of the express and most important offices of the lungs and skin is to carry them out of the body" (119).

This matter, if insufficiently dispersed, is taken back into the same (or another contingent) body, immersing it in its wastes instead of carrying them away: "the blood takes up with avidity all substances, even the most deadly poisons, when brought in contact with it in the form of a gas. . . . Any kind of noxious matter . . . is greedily sucked up by and mingled with the blood [through the lungs], and with that fluid it rapidly circulates and reaches all parts of the body" (121).[9] So much for the body's interior. In fact, one sees in medical theory by the 1860s a preoccupation with the body as surface, the emergence of the view of the body as multiple systems, and an overriding concern with bodily wastes. Intake is characterized not so much in terms of type and quantity as of purity, and the ability to distance one's body from excreta becomes crucial. The lungs and intestines are described as covered by a kind of skin continuing the permeable skin outside the body ("a skin without and a skin within, a covering skin and a lining skin," as one pamphlet put it), thus transforming the entire body into one surface, to which all was exterior, but entirely permeable. Having explained that the skin is full of "little invisible holes," the pamphlet continues,

> You will readily admit that three millions of holes and twenty-eight miles of pipes, are not likely to have been placed in the skin of a single body, without a purpose. . . . they are DRAINS AND SEWERS WHICH THE GREAT BUILDER, WHO MADE THIS HOUSE FOR YOU TO DWELL IN, HAS FURNISHED for carrying waste matter away from it. . . . **A quarter of an ounce of [decaying] poison is drained away** thorough the sewers of the skin, every day. (Ladies Sanitary Association 25–26, original emphasis)

Here the language of the clergy—of God's natural laws—is put to work in the sanitary project, and the analogy between body and built environment illustrates the focus on sanitation as control of the built environment—the

9. See also Henry Roberts, "Home Reform," dealing at length with similar issues.

bodies of inhabitants are to be disciplined to mirror the logical design of their dwelling places. The exteriorized practice of expert knowledges (sanitary architecture, urban design) are to be interiorized and practiced by the citizen.

Whereas the term "nuisance" was first used to refer to the accumulation of odorous wastes, by the 1860s those are considered secondary effects. (This is partly, of course, because measures to control nuisances had already been put into place.) As ever, the debate over powers to enforce the eradication of nuisances came into conflict with the interests of property, and it is significant that the costs of housing and landlord's rights to multiply rent were at issue in this debate, developing concurrently with reform debates intent on pricing respectability through rent levels. Such a debate took place during the Health of Towns deliberations in 1866, and the definition of overcrowding offered then is instructive. Radical MP for Tower Hamlets Acton Smee Ayrton read from the proposed bill the following definition: "'Any house, or part of a house, so overcrowded as to be dangerous, or prejudicial to the health of the inmates'" and asked, "what constituted the nuisance—the inmates or the house?" His colleague, Henry Austin Bruce, responded, "the nuisance was neither the house nor the inmates, but the overcrowding. . . . The physical evil [is bad, but worse are] the effects upon the morality of the people. In every large town thousands of persons were brought up in a state of moral degradation, which could only end in a great national danger" (*Hansard's* 182, Jul. 27, 1866: 1648). Here overcrowding (the cause) becomes the nuisance itself, as opposed to the effect.

The insistence on eradicating overcrowding focused on the homes rather than the workplaces of the working classes.[10] Often those urban workers whose dwellings and workplaces were separate were hardly in their "homes" except to sleep, but domesticity is the marked characteristic of the mid-century middle classes, whose supervision of the poor implied that their lives also should center on a separate and sacred domestic space. This is parallel to the gendering of domestic space at the middle-class level and its separation from the economic domain; if a separate domestic space is required to produce the social, then domesticity itself must be produced. Requiring a private space, clearly demarcated from public space, and often with multiple rooms at different levels of retirement from visitors, the domestic ideal encouraged the disaggregation of the mass.[11] Workers would be less mobile and more "steady," it was argued, if they had such a space to return to after work. The practical result of the rental qualification for the franchise was that to show "fitness,"

10. Sweatshops are sometimes the exception to this general trend.

11. Interestingly, in setting definitions for the 1866 Health Act, it was argued that a single family, no matter how large, could not overcrowd a dwelling; only the presence of multiple families or non–family members would do so.

a worker had to procure such a domestic space, thus showing not only economic means but the inculcation (incorporation?) of an appropriate desire.

Both poor environment and disease itself were held to have bad effects on massed bodies that would also affect the body social. Disease attacked persons, but the moral effects of disease were deleterious to populations. Chadwick and Smith argue, "Depression is the normal condition of the residents in all unhealthy districts. . . . The offspring of people in this enfeebled condition are puny and sickly . . . and the physical deterioration goes on increasing with each successive generation. . . . [This deterioration] is both more powerful and more constant than that produced by the most devastating wars." Further, by reducing the proportion of working adults to children and the aged in a population, "this destruction of the heads of family produce[s] . . . pauperism." Not only does the community then suffer economically but also morally, as "the steadying principle of the community is lessened, the acquisition of productive skill is obstructed, the difficulty of extending moral culture and forming moral habits is increased. . . . There is substituted a population always young, inexperienced, ignorant, credulous, passionate, violent, and proportionately dangerous, with a perpetual tendency to moral as well as physical deterioration" (Chadwick and Smith, 608–9). The rhetoric of fitness is in play here, as epidemics, according to Chadwick and Smith, create a population that is the very definition of the pauper mass (credulous, violent, without moral culture, unskilled, and undisciplined); crowding is the enemy of citizenship.

Crowding and unsanitary environments also were thought to create racial degeneration. In 1852 William Farr, Collator of Abstracts for the Registrar General's Office, wrote that

> the history of the nations on the Mediterranean, on the plains of the Euphrates and Tigris, the deltas of the Indus and the Ganges, and the rivers of China, exhibits this great fact—the gradual descent of races from the high lands, their establishment on the coasts in cities sustained and refreshed for a season by immigration from the interior; their degradation in successive generations under the influence of the unhealthy earth, and their final ruin, effacement, or subjugation by new races of conquerors. The causes that destroy individual men, lay cities waste which in their nature are immortal, and silently undermine eternal empires. ("Influence of Elevation" 174)

Farr thus provides a neat justification for imperialism, as well as staking Britain's racial claims to leadership on its public health and its geography. He explains that cholera is God's warning that the British community is also in danger of this elevation-related degeneration because so many have settled near the Thames: "the pestilence speaks to nations, in order that greater calamities than the death of the population may be averted. For to a nation of good and noble men Death, is a less evil than the Degradation of Race" (ibid., 178). Britain, however, Farr explains elsewhere, produces most of its population from high and salubrious areas; as for the rest, it could be fixed: "With wealth, industry and science at command, it is still possible to drain, and supply with pure water and a purer air, districts such as Southwark, Westminster, Liverpool and Hull" (*Mortality* xcviii). This improvement was not just a matter of correcting these defects, however, but of fostering human development toward perfection by restoring people to a natural environment: "let these human sacrifices suffice. The great Sanatory Reforms which will shield the country from pestilence, while they save the lives of thousands, will prevent the degradation of successive generations; and promote the amelioration and perfection of the human race" (ibid.).

The classes at issue in the second reform debate and in the sanitarians' labors were not, at least in public discourse, clearly defined. They were certainly measured, observed, and quantified to within an inch of their lives, but for most of the public, they were "the masses," "the million," "the residuum," the "dangerous classes," which might, depending on the context of the utterance, include (for example) manual laborers, or exclude them and oppose them to paupers per se. Although the pauper was the icon by which the negative aspects of the lower classes were signally represented, the lower laboring classes were precisely that grey area between the paupers, who were clearly outside the social body, and that body itself. Economically crucial and politically marginal, the working classes were socially liminal in this period, and it is exactly in that liminality that their danger lies. The well-fed, well-groomed, modest body (insulated in its 700-cubic-foot cushion of air), upright and manly, a little repulsed by the proximity of others, taking in its food alone, reading its individual newspaper, hungering for larger quarters with more separate rooms, more privacy, is the body of the citizen. The ill-fed, spindly, diseased, naked, dirty, "huddled masses" of pauperism, sharing sex, food, wastes, and political opinions indiscriminately in basements—and, it is argued, preferring it that way—is the anticitizen.

Social management is about management of the body, its health, morbidity, mortality, fertility, and waste—what goes into the body and what comes out of it. Political economy subsumes the economic problem of the laboring body/commodity into the larger context of resource management as a moral, as well as fiscal, issue, superimposing the individual body on the metaphor of the social body as it assimilates the economic unit of the family to that of a patriarchal state. T. H. Marshall, mid-century optimist, believed that citizenship would eventually abolish the inequities of social class; Bryan Turner has more recently modified that thesis to argue that "the dynamic feature of capitalism is precisely the contradiction between politics and economics as fought out in the sphere of social citizenship" (12).

I would add to that the observation that capitalism has dealt with this contradiction precisely by constituting the body of the subject in such a way that health and education, long understood as capital in their own right, have become a special part of the technology of consumption that enables the identity of the subject in the realm of the social. I mean by this that it is through (in this case) his own and his family's consumption—of housing, groceries, medical care, soap, and so on—that the subject constitutes his individual body as an acceptable part of the social body, as a citizen. It is the discourse of the sanitary movement that both constructs the social as body and "incorporates" the worker within the social—hence the language of reform debates, wherein the tropes of sanitation and urban planning become the grounding of definitions of citizenship. As the century progressed and early sanitary goals—the removal of dung heaps and installation of sewerage—were achieved, public health began to turn toward more direct behavioral modification as well as changes to the built environment. In the next section, we will take a closer look at the construction of the social as a separate domain and consider some examples of how a particular technology of social outreach—housing—became a forum for a feminized formulation of citizenship as homemaking.

SECTION II

Producing the Public: Public Health in Private Spaces

4

THE PUBLIC, THE PRIVATE, AND THE SOCIAL

> [T]he nuisance was neither the house nor the inmates, but the overcrowding. . . . The physical evil [is bad, but worse are] the effects upon the morality of the people. In every large town thousands of persons were brought up in a state of moral degradation, which could only end in a great national danger.
>
> —Mr. Bruce, *Hansard's,* July 27, 1866, 1648

Under the aegis of sanitary reform begun in response to epidemic diseases, public health, which came to include statistical monitoring of physical and what we would consider moral issues relating to matters of the public weal, became an important part of governing the social body at mid-century. When we speak of public health, we usually think of medicine practiced in the service of the public, often state supported, if not state implemented. This vague notion of a public is related to the sense of a "public" in Habermas's use of the term: a public formed of citizens in whose service the state labors and to whom it is accountable. Habermas states that "The line between state and society . . . divided the public sphere from the private realm" (30); it is that line between state and society, or more specifically, that realm of practices known as the social, with which we are concerned.[1] The social is an area technically associated with the "private" in the strict sense, but which actually

1. It is important to remember that Habermas chronicles the history of an ideal (though he himself sometimes appears to forget that), not an actual cultural structure. The distinction between the public and private spheres, which imaginatively structured social and political life in this period, was widely admitted and probably nowhere coherently practiced. (Amanda Vickery has famously charted the follies of too-literal interpretations of this division.) Also, the fantasy of an ideal public sphere is, throughout Habermas, shadowed by its less savory but more interesting twin, public opinion in an increasingly literate and powerful populace. The public sphere of Habermas's coffeehouses bears the relation to public opinion of the good citizen to the unreasoning mass of the mob. Although public opinion is not inherently and necessarily a degraded form of public communication, Habermas suggests that it can realize its proper form only under conditions that have never existed.

mediates between the shifting boundaries of public and private, in order to safeguard and produce that very split, in the service of the developing liberal conception of citizenship. The preceding chapters traced the specifically political discourse of fitness for citizenship and the developments of its investments in the private and domestic, that which would come to be understood as the domain of the social. This chapter is devoted to a detailed analysis of the stakes of the social and discussion of the current theoretical conversation on its status. In particular, I will be extending Mary Poovey's work on the social, which is foundational for this project. In examining the relation of public medicine to the social, we can interrogate the notion of a bourgeois public sphere and see how it depends on forms of panoptic oversight of the so-called private to secure the conditions of its possibility.

Public and Private

In the nineteenth century public medicine, or sanitary science, generally was conceived as a way of containing the spread of disease. The public it served was, early in the century, elite and bourgeois, and later, a public of largely bourgeois and bourgeois-aspirant citizens; the portion of the population on whom public medicine was actually practiced was outside this public. Initially, this target population was perceived as a permanently marginal group to be contained and managed, but by mid-century the continued existence of this group as such was seen as a failure of the public. The target group was, by the 1850s and 1860s, to be brought within the pale if possible, and this necessitated a different approach to public medicine: holistic and prophylactic rather than specific and ameliorative.

By the mid-nineteenth century, as is well known, private had come to refer to two areas: the domestic (what Habermas calls the intimate sphere) and the economic rights of private property. These were closely related; just as the nuclear family was often held in this period to be the basic unit of society and to mirror appropriate models of authority (benevolent paternalism), so was the economic freedom of the head of the family to be exercised in the interest of the family, and hence in the interest of the community, which was figured as an aggregate of families. The relationship of private to public in these two areas can be summarized as follows: family versus nonfamily; intimacy versus business; home versus street; home economics versus political economy; the economic (as a domain) versus the political; private property versus public obligation (or rights versus duties).

Hanna Pitkin asserts that "utilitarianism not only favored the representation of persons, but made interest an increasingly personal concept" ("Representation" 145).[2] Obviously, this model could be and was contested at the time; still, it remained the dominant model in popular understandings of political economy, and it reflected the liberal formula that only an atomized, economically independent subject could or would properly participate as a citizen of a liberal state. The domain of the public, on the other hand, had to do with the public weal and business of state. A casual glance at these distinctions reveals their tenuous quality. Habermas clarifies, "The sphere of the market we call 'private'; the sphere of the family, as the core of the private sphere, we call the 'intimate sphere.' The latter was believed to be independent of the former, whereas in truth it was profoundly caught up in the requirements of the market" (55–56). He also observes that the subjectivity explored and celebrated within the public sphere was one profoundly shaped by and dependent upon the hegemony of the nuclear family. I would add that this was the nuclear family experienced in a certain way: within a particular practice of domestic space with carefully mediated levels of publicity and seclusion, both within and from the immediate family. This model demanded multiple rooms and a certain amount of space devoted to the enactment and display of privacy.

Privacy on Display

As Elizabeth Langland has argued, Victorian domestic privacy itself had to be displayed, open to inspection ("Enclosure Acts" 8); bourgeois privacy, as an index of respectability, was also the visible representation of having *nothing to hide.* The absolute distinction between public and private, family and guests, and then again between inside and outside, allowed for a "social life" supposedly divorced from business and politics but in reality deeply embedded within them. Langland observes, "The [bourgeois country] house metaphorically and metonymically stood for power and one's moral entitlement to that

2. J. A. W. Gunn argues that Bentham is an exception and that, especially by the nineteenth century, "some of the factors that had once served to render intelligible talk of a sum of interests were no longer available. Natural rights played no great role in British political vocabulary. . . . Nor was the language of class conducive to visualizing the convergence of individual ambitions on a single range of conditions, such as those perceived as securing private rights" (204). He cites Mill's statement that individuals had both private interests and different "community interests" (206) as evidence that the Utilitarians were not so naïve on the topic as is often assumed. Indeed, this was hotly contested, but the dominant model of liberalism and laissez-faire was indeed dependent, at least in the popular understanding, if not in that of political scientists, on a notion of the identification of individual interests with the state. It is precisely this model that pitted citizenship against class in 1867, and which at last carried the second Reform Bill.

power. Because it operated most effectively through its continual visibility, it was thus open to random visitors and even its most intimate spaces could be penetrated with impunity" (ibid., 7–8). This "public privacy" depended heavily on the performances of women: "at the center of that visible structure stood the lady of the house, whose motions were precisely regulated by etiquette practices . . . that put her continually on display . . . the maintenance of wealth and power demanding continual visibility; continual visibility justifying the penetration of even private spaces; and private space gendered feminine so that the woman who is most protected by the architecture is also most exposed by it" (ibid.). Karen Chase and Michael Levenson's *Spectacle of Intimacy* also explores precisely this dynamic: increasing anxiety about intimacy becoming spectacle wherein the inviolate space of familial privacy was laid open through sensation novels and journalism. As they point out, however, it is crucial also to see in this "the extent to which domestic life itself was compelled toward acts of exposure and display" (7).

This display of privacy was enacted within an intermediate public of social peers and near peers, within which intimate-public processes (like friendly business) were conducted, and which was conceived as representative of the larger public realm. The much-vaunted privacy of the upper-middle-class family, therefore, was precisely the setting for semipublic rituals of visiting, dinners, at-homes, and so forth, conducted and overseen largely by women, which provided the vital stage upon which respectability might be displayed, power consolidated, alliances forged, courtships conducted. The division between public and private—politics and business, market and domesticity—had first to be consolidated for its erosion to be socially meaningful. Therefore, that division was sacred, precisely because its violation was so important to processes of meaning construction. The social, in the larger sense, was the domain of "society" in which the boundaries of the public and private were produced and policed. In the sense of social work and social intervention with which we shall largely be concerned here, it consisted of producing those distinctions where they did not exist or were inadequately or idiosyncratically inscribed.

The existence of the public required that of the private, defined against it. In the mid-Victorian period an elite quasi-public developed that mediated this dualism within which the social life of the middle classes and elites was enacted. The Habermasian public sphere of journalism commented on the elite performative public of representative government, which in turn, as reported in newspapers and *Hansard's,* came to exist as theatrical performance. This performance was increasingly directed at manipulating a mass public even as it purported to become more open and accessible to all members of the public through franchise reform. An intermediate and exclusive arena of debate and negotiation in which policy was made, conducted in clubs and in homes (at dinner parties, etc.), became ever more central to the operation of power even as it became less obvious that it was where power was located. Over the course of the mid-century, one sees in *Hansard's* an increasing sense of public attention to reporting: for example, MPs began to quote both newspapers and *Hansard's* in their speeches. This practice increased throughout mid-century and by the late 1860s was very well established, whereas in the 1830s MPs rarely cited such authorities. Their more frequent references to how the public, or publics composed of certain classes, would respond to certain parliamentary speeches or reporting of parliamentary activity also illustrates awareness of public opinion and of Parliament, as reported by the press, as a theater for the formation of public opinion and as an object of a broad public scrutiny and interpretation.[3]

In short, MPs showed an increasing awareness that an important role of parliamentary discourse was simply being reported in the mass press and that debates had to be managed for political effect upon that readership. The public opinion of the political elite and its hysterical shadow, the public opinion of the masses, were slowly becoming one in the understanding of elites.[4] Thus there emerged a further split between the public sphere performatively invoked during parliamentary debate and the kind of elite "public" sphere, based partially on a Habermasian principled argument and partially on the exigencies of realpolitik, which was conducted in behind-the-scenes negotiation between policy makers. In fact, the kind of public sphere that Habermas envisions in the late eighteenth century, which he notes was never fully realized even then, had become impossible even as it was cited as an ideal by the 1830s, with the expansion of the public and the accession of mass public opinion as a political force.

Additionally, there was always overlap between the critical commentary of "private persons" sufficiently influential to command a voice in the public sphere and the discourse of the state; many of these private persons had as much legislative power as MPs. One marker of the move away from even the

3. I should emphasize that the enactment of public politics as theatrical performance is hardly new in this period. My point is simply that the sense of the size and level of the audience, their direct political power, and their access to information—especially the privileged performance of parliamentary debate—changed dramatically over these thirty years.

4. Habermas discusses the use and distrust of "public opinion" as a kind of unreasoning public sphere in the nineteenth century. This, of course, is the mass public outside the elite. Although not a strong public in Nancy Fraser's sense, this was a public with a growing amount of political power, purchasing power, and, occasionally, brute force, one that overlapped with, but was not contained by, the bourgeois-elite sphere that had traditional strong public, that is, legislative, capability.

model of principled private citizens debating in open forum *in propria persona* was the move by some powerful journals, such as the *Edinburgh Review,* toward publication of unsigned articles, wherein opinion was represented as the preformed opinion of a certain public both constituted and represented by the journal rather than a private individual, an author (which Habermas's model requires). Thus, the spheres of political power, the public, and mass public opinion had more decisively split in Britain by this time than Habermas allows for.

The emergence of this intermediate public sphere in the political realm paralleled the habit of conducting business at home after dinner, or even the elaborate social rituals that supported business that would eventually be done elsewhere. (Today we might think of deal making on the golf course.) In the latter case, the parties took advantage of the partially spurious split between business and domesticity to conduct business in a less formal and often more effective way. Disraeli remarked that the half hour after dinner, in which gentlemen separated from the ladies of the house in order to drink and converse frankly, might well be the source of "the superiority of the English in political life in their conduct of public business and practical views of affairs" (*Coningsby* 109)—although, as we shall see, he also faulted the meddling of women in politics through "social influences." Perhaps this explains the ever-increasing differentiation of levels of privacy in the upper-middle-class home, as emerge in Victorian architect Robert Kerr's model of the gentleman's house: the absolute distinction between public and private, domestic and business, family and guests, allowing for a "social life" supposedly divorced from both business and politics but in reality intertwined with them. Of course, that "social life" was itself private and carefully policed to avoid too much openness of access to or contact with the larger world; strictly regulated visiting practices and the etiquette of introductions managed the apparently comparatively open flow of guests at, for example, a lady's at-home day. The existence of public opinion as mediated in journals, just like the existence of Parliament as theater, masked the uses of elite social life and lured with the promise of universal access to political power, through the franchise, and cultural power, through consumption.

The Social

The domain that mediated between public and private in order to create and sustain this division is what we have come to call the social.[5] Various theorists

5. Poovey and Jacques Donzelot place the earliest elaboration of the social in the late eighteenth

have placed the onset of the social at times ranging from the late 1700s to the early 1900s; Hannah Arendt famously found its emergence to be coterminous with the late modern period and the nation-state, and she believed that the social had utterly swallowed up both public and private, which then ceased to signify, leaving only a mass culture without a true possibility for individual freedom (28–41, and *passim*). However, if we time the elaboration of the social as the period in which it becomes possible to define it as both a field and a problem, that era comes to fruition in the nineteenth century. The social is perhaps most decisively inaugurated as a public and legislative issue in 1834, with the passage of the New Poor Law.[6] Arendt is quite right to argue that the social vexed the classical Aristotelian boundary between public and private, but it was far from abolishing the distinction. Instead, as we shall see, it reconstituted and protected that distinction, which, in the wake of an increasingly democratic political reformulation, required a new way to formulate the nature of the private and the political.

Society, in popular parlance, designated the arena of relations between and within (elite) families: friendship, courtship, and all the alliances on which business and community were based. The more specific use of the term "social" in this period is exemplified by its meaning in the Victorian phrase "social problems" and which we have come to associate with "social work": interventions into the lives of the poor, especially conceived as poor *families,* in order to correct problems largely thought to arise from inadequate socialization. The two uses are thus not unrelated; social work seeks to produce the values basic to society in a class that is seen as having insufficiently developed them.

Historians and theorists have had a good deal to say about the social, some of it contradictory. The most useful observations about the nineteenth century have been made by those working within a Foucauldian model, such as Poovey.[7] The divisions between the Habermasian tradition and the

---

century; others, such as Patrick Joyce and Nikolas Rose, have argued that the nineteenth century is largely a period before the social—certainly, if we define the social as Marshall does, in terms of rights, this is true. But for our purposes here, I will be defining it as a broader cultural phenomenon.

6. Jane Lewis has observed, "Social policies were only becoming matters of 'high politics' in the period 1870–1914" (3). This is indeed the case, because until the 1860s the social had not yet so visibly permeated all areas of economic and political life as to require institutionalization, which would serve to paradoxically strip it of a certain kind of authority derived from its separation from the political and economic, while at the same time legitimating its power—and to some extent that of feminism in this period—by institutionally validating the centrality of the social to the formation of the modern state. (Octavia Hill is right on the cusp of this transition, as we shall see.)

7. Rose situates the "invention of the social" at the beginning of the twentieth century (112), meaning that it was at this time that the emergence of social rights connected the social directly to the political in a new way—though I would say his own work indicates it is forming much earlier. Part of what I am doing here is providing the prehistory of that moment—and also complicating his

Foucauldian one are obviously deep. However, the ideal of the liberal public sphere discussed by Habermas was a powerful model in the nineteenth century. If we see *Structural Transformation* as a history of that never-realized vision, setting aside its nostalgia for a liberal universal subject, we can begin to see useful connections between the Foucauldian genealogies of the social and Habermas's elaboration of one of its most powerful enabling fantasies. I would like to synthesize some of the most useful and interesting work for our purposes, in order to elaborate some possibilities for understanding the relationship of the social to the public sphere and liberal governmentality.

Mary Poovey, who has given us the most richly provocative elucidation of the social body in the early Victorian period, places the development of the social in the late 1700s, allying it with the development of statistical and theoretical representations of populations as aggregates. This time period, according to Poovey, corresponds with the first clear sense of the social sphere as distinct from the domains of economics and politics:

> These two developments—the aggregation of distinct populations and the conceptual disaggregation of a social domain—were intimately connected, for identifying the problems that afflicted the nation involved isolating the offending populations, abstracting from individual cases the general problems they shared, and devising solutions that would not contradict the specific rationalities of those domains by which British social relations had traditionally been organized. (*Making* 8)

At the same time, Poovey notes, it was fundamental to "political rationality" that political power should be based in the ownership of property, even as it became increasingly widely believed that trade and commerce should be liberated from governmental interference. Therefore, the appearance of the social as a separate domain was associated with "the specification of a set of problems that was related to but not coincident with political and economic issues" (ibid.). By 1832, as we have seen, the move from property ownership to rental as the basis of the franchise was a significant step in a move to a capitalist understanding of the notion of the political stakeholder. This development eventually necessitated an ideal of universal inclusion, rather than simply of management or suppression of the excluded portion of the total population.

---

assumption that the connection to the political is "new" in this period. He follows Foucault in arguing that "the social" emerged in part out of the nineteenth-century concept of society as population, that is, as an organic whole subject to its own recognizable laws and capable of evolving or degenerating (115).

As we have also seen, citizenship—of a nation—was the notion of community explicitly counterpoised by Victorians to emerging class solidarity in this period. Citizenship and the bourgeois public sphere were seen as universal (or at least national) and were offered specifically as a form of identity that not only subsumed but also operated *against* class and other local identities with subversive potential, an ideal public that neutralized more potentially politically effective, if marginal, counterpublics.[8] But it was not necessary for Victorian liberalism to make the basis of political action itself the identity of citizenship, so long as personal and economic actions were conducted on that basis, which could itself be mystified as that of "society" or even "nature" rather than attributed to the aims of state. There are two issues here: political activism and a sense of public communitarian identity through what we often call "public spiritedness"; it is not so much the former as the latter that Victorians were concerned with inculcating in the nascent citizen. (As we will see, for example, it was precisely this sense of larger communitarian identity that housing activist Octavia Hill valued.) In this model, it was only when a clear distinction was made between "private identities" and public ones that successful entry into civil society was secured.

Habermas notes, "The same process that converted culture into a commodity . . . established the public as in principle inclusive. . . . It always understood . . . itself . . . within a more inclusive public of all private people . . . [who] could avail themselves via the market of the objects that were subject to discussion." Habermas admits that this idealized equality did not emerge in practice and also that this public was quite small (30). But this is an important point—Habermas considers the real problem with the bourgeois public sphere to be in its incomplete instantiation of reason as the basis of discourse and true universality of access; he sees the ideal as a good thing. However, the notion of universality is at heart inimical to the concerns of minority groups, which may often, with more political profit, form their own counterpublics.[9] It also mystifies the real inequalities of participants and

8. We still see this confusion operating today; for example, Michael Walzer notes that, certainly now, and even in the nineteenth century, public (political) identity usually forms a relatively small and marginal locus of identification and participation for most people. He attributes this to the competition of more local identities with that of citizenship in a complex society; local identities such as class and ethnicity, he argues, "separate and divide" people, making for "the primacy of the private realm" ("Citizenship" 218). Obviously, these identities only separate and divide a whole that is arranged on some more privileged basis; they can also be potent forces for community. It is, in short, a false dichotomy to set national citizenship as the only possible public identity against a wholly atomized and politically ineffectual "privacy."

9. Nancy Fraser observes that for Habermas, the class struggle fragmented the public sphere into competing groups. She argues, however, that this dialogue between interests is required for a true public sphere to exist.

distracts from the modes in which power may really be operating behind the scenes by perpetuating the illusion of transparency and access.[10] Habermas believes that it is precisely the ideal of such universality, through citizenship potentially available to all, that safeguards the bourgeois public sphere; it is not in that it is actually but *potentially* all-inclusive that its virtue lies. By the time this potential inclusiveness even begins to be an ideal, however, the eighteenth-century notion of a bourgeois public sphere is already being replaced by the less rational domination of a "mass" public opinion, distrusted by elites, who increasingly saw themselves in the role of its managers rather than informers.

I would argue that in fact, it is the articulation of the social, part of which is the identification of the so-called social problem, that opposed and masked difference. The social enacted precisely the fantasy of equivalence that the public sphere demands—that is, that economic inequality did not need to be addressed in order to have social and political equality of access. Therefore, the emergence of the public sphere was not "accidentally" undercut by the coincidental emergence of social problems; in fact, it emerged in order to manage those problems themselves. The construction of class conflict as a "social problem" is illustrative of this point. Class identification, when chosen over a more generalized social/national identification, was seen as problematic; amelioration of this conflict was geared toward eliminating the importance of class identification, not at easing class inequality of access to power (as we saw in the debates on the second Reform Bill). It was not simply liberalism but also capitalism that demanded the inclusion of the lower classes in public life in the nineteenth century,[11] and emerging understandings of the body confirmed that there was no insulation possible from the effects of an insufficiently interpellated constituency of the economic or sanitary body. Disease could leap class barriers, and undernourished infant bodies grew up to be inadequate workers and soldiers. The social was the realm through which all must pass to be properly interpellated.[12]

10. Geoffrey Eley notes that the bourgeois public sphere is, in fact, based on systematic exclusions.

11. I am making not a theoretical argument positing capitalism as a necessary condition of the public sphere but a historical observation about the dependency of emerging consumer capitalism in Britain on such a structure.

12. Mary Poovey has done the most to articulate the connections among the social, the economic, and the aims of liberal government, but problems of definition remain thorny when we try to widen the scope of her argument using her terms. She argues that the social is "related to but not coincident with" the economic and political (*Social Body* 8). Certainly, the political and economic are profoundly dependent on the social and produce the social in order to safeguard their own operations. The question of "disaggregation," as Poovey uses the term above to claim that the social disaggregates from other domains to form a new domain of knowledge, is evidently a complex one. In the sense that areas

Poovey claims that between the 1830s and 1850s, "we can see . . . the complete disaggregation of the social, and then its reformation in the very image of the economic. . . . By the 1850s, pauperism had disappeared as a problem, *not* because there were no poor people but because the social sphere, to which pauperism had been assigned, had come to *mirror* the economic domain, where individuals appeared as independent, self-regulating agents. (*Social Body* 11, her emphasis). But the social did not simply mirror the economic after the 1850s; the social formed in the split between politics, economics, and the moral domain. It did follow political economy in its insistence on independence and economic equivalence; however, its feminized status and maternalism were enacted as a phase in the development of the citizen: the citizen passes through the social, is socialized, by a properly domestic maternal figure in order that he will, in turn, behave economically so as to reproduce that ideal domestic environment, safeguarding the social. Paupers were not independent, self-regulating agents, which was precisely why they were to be brought through the social and retrained—remothered—so that they might someday enter the economic domain as self-regulating agents.

The social did not simply mirror the economic domain but mediated between that domain and that of the public, of citizenship. Yes, individuals appeared as self-regulating agents, but some persons' lack of training to be independent necessitated socialization in proper domesticity so that freedom could be rightly exercised for their own good and the good of the community: through being part of a family, one came to understand being part of a larger public community. In other words, individuality and self-regulation were not essential characteristics of persons; they had to be cultivated. The social provided both the matrix of formation of the separation between domains and the safety valve between them.

The Social and the Public-Private Divide

It is in the elaboration of this problem that Poovey might profitably be placed in dialogue with Habermas.[13] By examining the relationship between the

---

of community life that had previously been connected, through clerical authority and so forth, are both formalized and separated from other areas of practice, this is a good description. However, the term "disaggregation" might be read to imply a process involving an already existing set of *practices,* and this is in fact not the case. The social is produced as much as (or more than) "disaggregated"; it is a new phenomenon that subsumes some older practices, but it also integrates them in a new epistemological and economic framework in the service of an emerging political-economic model that in turn produces some wholly new practices as well.

13. Poovey dismisses the possibility: "The domains I have been discussing did not correspond to

social and the public-private distinction, and showing its operation in a few instances, I hope to demonstrate a vital connection between the domains described by Poovey and Habermas and to illustrate its operation in the service of liberal governmentality. The social produced, mystified, mediated, and monitored the split between public and private: it produced it by providing an arena in which privacy was performed; in so doing, it mystified the tenuous and unstable nature of the distinction; thus, it mediated between public and private by providing a "buffer domain" in which the shifting distinction could be continually elaborated and affirmed; and therefore it provided a stage upon which demonstrations of privacy could eventually be publicly monitored.

Scholars agree that the social was from the beginning gendered feminine, in part because of its investment in conceptions of affective, often familial and physical intimacy.[14] The social domain, associated with caretaking, child rearing, and the notion of sympathy as the affective glue that held the domain together, was resolutely connected to a feminine domestic epistemology. It is worth paying attention to where this epistemology was being constructed and found its authority. Nancy Armstrong has analyzed its history in this period at length in *Desire and Domestic Fiction.* She argues that by figuring men "no longer [as] political creatures so much as they were products of desire and producers of domestic life" (4), novels positioned women as individuals to be valued for their innate qualities of mind, cultivated by moral and sentimental education, which was directed at managing desire and inculcating sympathy. Although this development was key to the construction of separate (gendered) spheres, she avers, it apparently depoliticized the feminine and

---

either of the senses in which contemporaries used the categories of public and private spheres. Not only was the social a domain overseen by both governmental and private initiatives, but the boundary between the private (voluntary or domestic) and the public (governmental or market-related) was permeable (for some individuals more than others) in a way that did not exactly correspond to the permeability of the boundary between the social and political domains" (*Social Body* 12–13). The relationship between the social, on the one hand, and the public and the private, on the other, is one Poovey does not discuss further, largely because of the discontinuities she cites here, but the emergence of the social at the same time as the emergence of the ideal of the bourgeois public sphere as Habermas defines it should encourage us to seek connections. In short, Habermas admits the practical lack of realization of the ideal in this period but fails to account for both the ideal's efficacy in the social imaginary and its lack of full implementation, whereas Poovey elaborates the relation of the social to the development of mass culture under capitalism and the feminization of the social, but not the nature of its oddly interdependent yet discontinuous relationship with the political.

14. Denise Riley argues that the social is gendered feminine from the moment of its construction in its articulation of an emotional and moral standard for perception. She comments, "One striking effect of this conceptualizing of the 'social' is its dislocation of the political. The latter takes on an intensified air of privacy and invulnerability, of 'high politics' associated with juridical and governmental power in a restricted manner," which in turn restricts what can be defined as political (50–51).

sentiment in the service of "the economic triumph of the new middle classes" (10).[15] It might be useful here to think in terms of Nancy Fraser's concept of multiple publics in opposition to the dominant one, with varying degrees of "strength" (i.e., performative power), whose discourse interacts with the hegemonic public in various ways: supporting, modifying, opposing, and so on. Certainly, the moral authority of feminine sympathy and management of desire came at the cost of any site of direct political intervention. Interestingly, then, the domain of the social, which became a site of public address for these women, had to do with precisely sexuality, household management, and sympathy—putatively noneconomic, apolitical concerns mobilized precisely in the service of a particular economic and political model. Private persons as, in Habermas's phrase, "human beings pure and simple" were to be formed within and by domestic attachments, under the primary authority of the mother: it was this maternal figure who was the harbinger and ruler of the social. Yet this social tutelage prepared the young for the larger and related protocols of the public, the political, and the economic. Thus, the social mediated between the public and private but in a very particular way, in that the social prepared potential citizens for public life but essentially involved the regulation of the private: in the case of philanthropic or governmental social outreach, it involved domestic practices, individual economic practices, especially those related to domesticity, and the bodily practices of those individuals deemed to have an insufficient sense of proper private practice. Social surveillance and intervention produced and secured privacy in a class that did not practice it, so they could learn to value the distinction between public and private, which could be leveraged for social control and respectability.

We can trace here the Aristotelian model of citizenship and public life as that which transcends the concerns of the domestic sphere—the body's

15. This leads us to first question why the social was understood, as Poovey argues, as "work that could be seen as an extension of domestic offices" (43) in the first place: Poovey seems to imply that this was an accidental by-product of the construction of the social "in the image of the economic"; in fact, this femininity is quite central to the construction of the social as mediator. Poovey makes the same move with the social that Habermas makes with the public: Poovey sees the whole social domain as essentially homogenous instead of stratified in its own right (in this case, between analysis and intervention); Habermas sees the public sphere, comprising both political and literary discourse, as seamlessly intertwined, although he observes that individuals had differing levels of access to these two arenas of subject formation: "The circles of persons who made up the two forms of public were not even completely congruent. Women and dependents were factually and legally excluded from the political public sphere, whereas [they] . . . took a more active part in the literary public sphere. . . . Yet . . . in the self understanding of public opinion, the public sphere appeared as one and indivisible" (55–56). But we know that the areas of public, journalistic discourse were not homogenous in "public opinion" but were clearly demarcated in elaborate, if unstable, hierarchies. Literary discourse, especially Habermas's privileged form, the novel, was seen as inferior, suspect, feminine, and requiring careful discipline and surveillance throughout this period.

unceasing demands and the manipulation of household objects that demands the attention of the homemaker and caregiver. As Octavia Hill, who was to proudly claim her housing work as both feminized and private (that is, apolitical and anti-institutional), put it, "Not a small thing, even in itself, is the dealing with the tangible and soulless things of the earth. We may be very proud, justly proud, of the well-ordered spot of earth, the well-spent income, the self-restrained providence, whether they are our own, or whether we have helped another so to regulate the talents entrusted to him" (*Our Common Land* 44). But while one was concerned with the tangible and soulless things of the earth, one was pointedly not to be concerned with legislating the overarching structures into which they are "ordered." Social work was assimilated into household management and, by definition, away from politics per se. Once the spot of earth was thoroughly well ordered, probably by a housewife, then, perhaps, the owner of the well-spent income might look to public affairs.

It was this persistent gendering of a mind-body, public-domestic split that underlay the uneasy fit between capitalist notions of public fitness as connected to the production of a persona through material objects (the Gaian approach to citizenship) and an older, more aristocratic, notion of a subject essentially freed from such considerations. The contradiction in this position, of course—and it was one exploited by the middle classes to claim their own public identity—was that the aristocratic, Aristotelian model was still based on a notion of stakeholding tied to material wealth. It simply relied on a relationship to that wealth mediated by the feminine domestic manager (or effeminized servant class) to produce a masculine public identity free from such concerns.

As we have seen, citizenship, as membership in a universal social body, offering participation in the public sphere through the franchise and a public national culture through consumption, was counterpoised against local identities, especially class, in the 1860s. The concept of public well-being inherent in public medicine depended upon being able to monitor and assure proper private practices and enforce the distinction between the two. The lower working classes, however, just outside the borders of the social body, just beneath the minimal economic requirements required for the franchise, were worrisome precisely because they did not seem to practice a private form of domesticity: doing paid work in their domestic space, sharing sleeping quarters with non–family members or with those of the opposite sex, and so on. Social experts, pushing for house-to-house visitation and intervention, found themselves in the peculiar position of arguing that working-class privacy must be penetrated because it did not exist, or that proper privacy could only be learned under supervision. Middle-class women, the center of the domestic and social, must take working-class women under their tutelage, to enable them in turn to produce the social in their own domestic space.

Woman to Woman: Producing the Social

To the extent that the social was feminized—in part, that meant particularized instead of abstracted—it remained outside the political. In order for social information to be transformed into policy through the expert knowledges of biopolitics, it had to be generalized through statistics. Thus, the construction of the social at the legislative level required, as Poovey notes, a certain abstraction. However, biopolitical knowledges moved in two directions—the gathering of information and the use of that information, where abstract knowledges had to be, at least in part, reparticularized. The social as a field of practices (as opposed to knowledge), like the "two forms" of public sphere mentioned by Habermas, was stratified.[16] Social work, although indeed generally feminized, had two aspects, analysis and intervention, each of which worked on a real and metaphorical level in a polarized gender relationship: observation, analysis, and finally legislation by male administrators, often sanitarians; individual intervention by female and (feminized) male district visitors, clergy, and paid sanitary police.[17] When tutelary intervention became the norm, it was almost entirely practiced at mid-century by women and clergy—the "private," voluntary sector.[18] Although I agree that individuals exploited and resisted the construction of the social to a number of ends,

16. Poovey connects the construction of the social with a privileging of abstraction; she then argues that women such as Ellen Ranyard, who began the "Bible women" movement, were able to use the feminization of the social against abstraction and in the service of a more richly individualized understanding and intervention (27). However, this personal connection was based on what was thought to be (abstractly enough) a more or less universal feminine aptitude for personalizing and relating on a maternal basis (one might think of Romney Leigh's indictment of women as "hard to general suffering"). This was what made women such good social workers, the logic ran—and such bad politicians.

17. Seth Koven notes in his excellent study of same-sex desire and philanthropic work, "By the first decade of the twentieth century, two hierarchies were becoming rapidly entrenched. Men came to control sociology as an academic discipline while women dominated the supposedly more practical fields of social work and home economics" (*Slumming* 225). As we will see with Octavia Hill, this formulation is firmly rooted in mid-century developments.

18. Dorice Williams Elliott observes that the new form of the social "fell between" the public and private spheres and "blurred the boundaries between them" (113). She argues, correctly I believe, that although the social could be classified as public because of its connection with male professionals, its association with the family allowed women to be experts and opened the door for their professionalization. This process created competition between male and female experts for authority over the social sphere (114).

and that for middle-class women it was a realm that provided particularly empowering possibilities for identity construction and intervention, I think we have to be careful about "romanticizing resistance." The power of the social enabled liberal feminism eventually to make the moves it did; it also created some of the conditions that necessitated those moves in the first place.[19]

These assumptions about the separation of the social and the political operated at a sufficiently overt level that they could be identified and critiqued by those they were presumed to define. John Bright, the radical reformer, spoke to this in 1866. As Margot Finn points out, his rhetoric "broke new ground . . . by justifying democratic reform as an agent of social change" (251); more to our purposes here, it did so in part by refuting the claims of the feminized, apolitical social as a remedy to the ills of the class system. Bright argues that

> this mass of misery . . . is so great a mass that benevolence cannot reach it. . . . There does not exist among created beings, beneath the angelic ranks, those who are more kind and charitable than the women of the United Kingdom. But benevolence can touch scarcely the fringe of this vast disorder. . . . Justice is impossible from a class. It is most certain and easy from a nation. . . . If class has failed, let us try the nation. That is our faith, that is our purpose, that is our cry—let us try the nation. (Ibid., 251)

G. W. M. Finn has shown how, after the failure of the Charter, radicals such as James Bronterre O'Brien and Reynolds turned to a vision that refused to separate political and social spheres, insisting on social rights and reforms, including universal education, because they believed that no true political transformation was possible without a social transformation preceding it

19. Frank Prochaska's very useful book on nineteenth-century philanthropy makes the related point that women's philanthropic activities prepared them over the course of the century for entry into the public sphere, especially the campaign for women's suffrage, toward the end of the period—a point with which I basically concur. Here, however, I am interested in clarifying this complex trajectory, which necessitates understanding the relationship between public, private, and social, on which Prochaska does not elaborate. This relationship is crucial to understanding why, in Prochaska's view, women such as Hill and Ranyard were, as a contemporary critic charged, too interested in the social and not in what he calls "theory" (133)—that is, public issues such as political economy. Prochaska attributes the lack of such interest to a "pragmatic, unanalytic mentality encouraged in the other spheres of their lives," which discouraged them from being interested in such abstract concepts (134). On the contrary, I would say that Hill, for example, had a rather comprehensive theory about the organization of the social body and its relationship to nation, as I discuss in chapter 6. It is the explicit connection of that to political economy and politics which she regards as outside the appropriate feminine sphere of the social and, indeed, antithetical to it. It is impossible to understand this disconnect without also understanding the vexed relationship of the social to the mid-Victorian public sphere, as well as the two-tier stratification of the social mentioned above.

(ibid., 86–87). These radicals used for their own purposes the rhetoric of elites who first posed nation as a safe alternative to class identity. We see in this stance the early recognition that the social and political were falsely separated in Britain, as well as the acceptance of the social as occupying a maternalist position vis-à-vis the politically aware citizen.

Women were ultimately responsible for the social (or antisocial) behavior of both children and husbands, despite having little legal authority. The woman, with the help of various social professionals, including the clergy, medics, philanthropists, and, later, schools, was finally responsible for mobilizing her family's consent to social prohibitions.[20] It was up to the woman to take responsibility for creating a domestic environment that would inculcate proper social and economic behavior on the part of the husband and children. And to model this behavior, who better than a woman already properly socialized? In Britain the model of "ladies' philanthropy" and religious visiting under clerical supervision provided an existing structure for the transition to visiting for more secular purposes.

It has been observed that citizenship under liberal government involves the mobilization of consent—you have perfect freedom to do what you want to do so long as you want to do what everyone else does. Privacy is located in personal economic affairs and in the domestic sphere, wherein, it is assumed, if one behaves "naturally," one will act in the most beneficial economic manner: that is, produce an appropriately sized nuclear family and save money to safeguard and improve that family's future, improvement being defined as more space, more privacy, proper adherence to bourgeois gender roles, and so on. However, as the working classes commanded more purchasing and political power in the mid-century, it became evident that they could not be relied upon to behave "naturally." Just as personal economic affairs became more liable to scrutiny as the century progressed, and as desirable economic behavior was rewarded with citizenship (e.g., the franchise), anxiety about domestic behavior was rising.[21]

20. As Donzelot notes, "Housing had to become a factor that complemented the school in the supervision of the children: . . . The search for intimacy and the domestic jurisdiction that was proposed to the working-class woman were the means to make this dwelling acceptable and even attractive, in the transition from a schema that was tied to production and social life to a conception based on separation and surveillance. If the husband preferred the outside . . . and the children the street . . . this would be the fault of the wife and mother" (44–45).

21. Privacy and its display became a matter of obsessive concern in the mid-century. In the 1860s the tension between visibility and invisibility was exploited by sensation novels, in which the middle-class home veils a dark secret. It is worthy of note that the sensation plot often exposes a lower-class woman in the upper-class home, whose inadequate sexual privacy creates a scandal: *Lady Audley's Secret* comes to mind. The middle class's increasing seclusion, recast in terms of class conflict, became the locus of fantasies of murder and rape (most dramatically illustrated in the W. T. Stead exposés at

The mid-century sanitary movement's attention focused on the built environment. In part, of course, it emphasized fostering cleanliness; in larger part, it embraced the notion of caring for, educating, and managing the poor family so that they might be brought within the social body. The social body overlapped with the body politic (especially from the 1860s on),[22] but it exceeded it in the sense that it contained and indeed primarily depended upon women and children. It was also discontinuous with it in the sense that the social *produced* both public and private—citizen and family member and *homo economicus*—but was itself regarded as divorced from the economic and political, instead having its heart in the domestic, the intimate, and the moral. It was profoundly feminized and identified with the results of successful domestication/domesticity. However, it was connected to and overseeable by those technicians of the social, public medics: sanitary reformers, sanitary police, and boards of health. It was the "scientific" status of these experts that legitimated their apparent disconnection from the contingencies of politics and economics. It was these experts' vital connection to the maternal (legitimated as "nature") in caring for health and morality that enabled them to claim a cultural authority mobilized in the service of universal inclusion in the liberal state through indoctrination into proper domestic habits. These habits were believed to demand and, indeed, to generate proper hygienic and economic behavior. The cost of this apparent disassociation from the economic and political was perhaps partially evidenced in England's inability to pass any health or housing legislation with real teeth until late in the century. As we shall see, this split temporarily resolved itself in the tiering of the social into a masculinized institutional policy and feminized philanthropic outreach. As we shall also see, the sheltering of social outreach in the feminized domestic domain became increasingly difficult to sustain.

---

the end of the century, wherein the relative retirement of the middle-class urban house's inner rooms was read as a site for sadistic sexual abuses). The lower working classes, however, appeared to lack private domesticity, engaging in an obscene, rather than an appropriate, transparency.

22. It should be clarified that we are talking here about the social imaginary. In fact, of course, the 1867 bill did not enfranchise many urban working-class men—and never aimed, even in its most progressive moments, at the enfranchisement of more than a relatively small number of fairly well-off skilled laborers. But it was widely *believed* that respectable working-class enfranchisement was the issue at stake in this reform, and that belief created a far more progressive vision than the actual bill had any relation to.

5

HOUSING THE SOCIAL BODY

> Having "a room of one's own" is a desire, but also a control.
>
> —Gilles Deleuze, on Jacques Donzelot

Housing and Sanitary Reform

The operations of the social, as we have seen, were rooted in the domestic sphere. Nowhere did domesticity and the authority of the state come into clearer contact than in the sanitary movement and its important subfield, housing reform. By the 1860s housing reform came to be one of the chief means of sanitary intervention. The housing crises of the nineteenth and early twentieth centuries, like the development of public medicine, are characteristically understood as exemplifying the conflict between laissez-faire economic policy and decentralized government, and the centralization of authority, necessary to industrialism, that was spurred by contagious diseases and increasing medical knowledge. The fear of disease was a principal motive in housing reform. In his 1850 treatise on cholera, medic and scientist John Stevenson Bushnan observes that it is the condition of the homes of the poor that gave the epidemic he is discussing its particular virulence, musing, "To most persons the very name of 'home' has associated with it some of the tenderest reminiscences; but how sad the reflection that the poor man's home should be infested with all the elements of disease and death!" (37). Bushnan here appeals to the ideology of domesticity—how can the poor develop a proper sense of domestic identity in a home associated with disease? He moves to a Kingsleyan appeal to cross-class sympathies—and underscores it with the threat of cross-class vulnerability:

> In passing through London, the most superficial observer cannot fail to notice that the squares and streets are built with a scrupulous regard to the

> different ranks of society. The courtly part of the metropolis is distinct from the commercial; while in each we can descend from broad thoroughfares, flanked on each side by well-built houses, to narrow lanes, squalid courts, and filthy alleys. . . . The mechanic, who has wages to afford it, occupies the respectable back street; in the next, the labourer, with more limited means; while thieves, beggars and prostitutes take refuge in the various "rookeries" open for their reception:
>
> I turned from an alley 'neath the wall,
> And stepp'd from earth to hell!—The light of Heaven,
> And common air was narrow, gross and dim;
> The tiles did drop from the eaves; the unhinged doors
> Totter'd o'er inky pools, where reek'd and curdled
> The offal of a life.
> Shrill mothers cursed; wan children wailed; sharp coughs
> Rang through the crazy chambers; hungry eyes
> Glared dumb reproach, and old perplexity,
> Too stale for words; o'er still and webless looms
> The listless craftsmen through their elf-locks scowl'd.
> (Bushnan 38)

Not only does the physical environment of these "homes" threaten to disintegrate—tiles dropping, doors unhinged and hanging open—but the residents themselves are liquefying into "inky pools"—the "offal of a life"—before our eyes. Both the chambers and the inhabitants are "crazy" and "perplexed." The working men are "listless" and unproductive, following on (and from) women who mother badly. And of course the sewage in the center of the street refers us directly to the threat of disease, also indicated by the chorus of coughs. The shift in tone and mode of narration (from straightforward description to quoted poetry) mirrors a common shift in treatises that describe the homes of the very poor: either the narrator will resort to literary references, often Miltonic, or to fanciful metaphors, or to a simple declaration of the inability of narrative to adequately convey the horror of the homes and surroundings he is describing. In this text narration takes us through all social levels to the rookeries, populated by the underclass, which only then necessitates a shift in mode of discourse. The living conditions of the very poor frustrated narration in the scientific form of the sanitary report, even while such reports existed mostly to describe these indescribable circumstances. In this way the excess and filth of the city continually threatened to exceed the bounds of the scientific processes developed to define them, rendering them opaque (indescribable, incomprehensible) rather than transparent to the gaze of the reformer.

In addition to the cholera epidemics that began calling attention to the depredations of disease in slum areas as early as 1832, the flight of middle-class residents from the urban core, along with the concentration of work and workers in the high-priced central regions, precipitated a crisis, both of space availability and of runaway profiteering by landlords and speculative builders. Housing historian Richard Rodger identifies two labor practices that had a serious impact on workers' housing: the practice of hiring by the day or half day, which made living close to the workplace essential, and the "rhythm of work itself," with its meal breaks ideally—and cheaply—taken at home. But, Rodger also points out, the workers' proximity to the workplace "meant competition with industrial, retailing and commercial land uses. . . . Rents formed a disproportionately high percentage" of workers' expenses (12).

Sanitary Desire

Contemporary analyses of this phenomenon, even by sympathetic observers, show the difficulty of Victorians in mediating between a rhetoric of economic determinism and one of individual responsibility. Edward Gotto, inspector for the Commissioners of Sewers, was clearly able to understand the economics of the system and place the blame on the owners and the faulty reforms of earlier years, which pulled down slums without considering where the displaced population would go. In discussing the slums of St. Giles, he gives the reader a sense of the stakes of such an error in judgment, describing infant mortality rates of up to nearly half of all children under the age of two, which was double the mortality rate of Lambeth, another fairly poor parish. He also points out that "reforms" that consisted of pulling down overcrowded properties simply created even worse overcrowding as displaced tenants flocked to the remaining buildings and rents were driven even higher for less space (6). He gives detailed descriptions of the economic arrangements of each of the offending properties, noting that they were owned by upper-class landlords and divided and subleased through so many intermediaries that these foul slums produced the highest rents of any real estate in the city. One property in St. Giles, "the resort of the most depraved and filthy class of the community," operated this way: "Two or three houses are underlet to a lessee for a term of years, at about 20L per annum; he underlets the property house by house at about 35L per annum; these are again let out in rooms at a still greater remunerative rent; and lastly, the separate beds in rooms are underlet to vagrants, tramps, and the refuse of society, at about 3d. per night; producing, after deducting rates, taxes, and losses, about 70L. per house per annum." The sanitary conditions of such property were predictably appalling: "So large a number of houses having been destroyed, the consequent crowded state of this spot is scarcely credible. . . . Many of the houses originally had privies, but they were destroyed by the sub-landlords for the purpose of avoiding the enormous periodical cost of emptying the cesspools." In this neighborhood "110 persons, sleeping in three houses, are compelled to use the necessary in another street" (1–4).

Gotto avoids resorting to the muse to describe this neighborhood; instead, he insists on the inability of prose to depict the situation upon which he was, after all, sent to report: "No adequate description can convey the horrors and depravity pervading this place; and instead of occupying the Commissioners' time with details too disgusting for expression, I would rather proceed with the development of a plan." Strikingly, despite the fact that he has earlier in a four-page span recorded the complaints of people living in these dwellings about their cleanliness and noted that these people would accept sanitary help if they could get it, he concludes that the cause of all this crowding is the inappropriate desire of the tenants: "Under any other circumstances such property would not realise a rent of more than L10. per annum at the most. I am led to believe the present value is caused by the propensity of this class of persons to congregate together, and so create a demand" (ibid.).

Even after Gotto analyzes the economic conditions that have led to the degradation of the slums, he takes refuge in a consumerist model. Though the tenants complain and want better conditions, he reasons, since such property, under *normal* conditions, could not generate so much wealth, it must be the "propensity of this class of persons to congregate" that has created a demand. In short, it is the unnatural desires of the residents that have created the situation from which upper-class slumlords realize their profits. Some of this same ambivalence can be seen in General Board of Health doctor John Sutherland's description of disease in the same area, which draws, in part on Gotto's report: "Cholera and Diarrhoea have been very prevalent within the last fortnight in the neighborhood of Church-lane. . . . The occupants have complained sadly for some time of the stench arising from the drain. . . . The locality is both confined and unhealthy, from the dirty habits of the Irish who frequent it, and the drainage of the houses and the ventilation of the sleeping-rooms very imperfect" (4). Even though the inhabitants have complained, apparently unavailingly, Sutherland is inclined to see the habits of the Irish tenants as at least as much to blame as the inadequate water supply and sewerage. In his description of an adjacent building, we see the same logic: "The whole structure and arrangement of the dwellings is about as bad as can be conceived, and they appear to have attracted towards them some of the worst classes of the population in the metropolis. It is the result of observation, that if dwellings be ever so bad, there will still be people found of a character similar to the dwellings to inhabit them" (5–6). Shortly thereafter he returns to this theme, attempting to account for the "attractiveness" of such rentals: "Unhealthy localities attract certain classes of people, and overcrowding renders cleanliness and ventilation very difficult, even if the people were disposed to put them into operation. Unhealthy houses act upon the people, and the people re-act upon the houses, and thus cause and effect are interchanged, and the result is disease mortality, demoralization and crime" (6).

The structure requires remediation, not only because it makes it difficult for the residents to develop good habits but also because it "attracts"—indeed, creates—consumers of "a similar character" to the physical structure. There is, obviously, little recognition in Sutherland's statement of the economic necessities and pricing strategies that make this lodging so "attractive." Still, there is a troubled sense that one cannot quite decide where exactly the blame should go. The buildings and the tenants create each other; since modifying people directly is difficult, the more docile built environment should be submitted to the "remedies required," which will then "act upon the people." Sutherland concludes this section of the report by again quoting Inspector Grotto's report on this slum's overcrowding of "'all ages and both sexes . . . herded together with a proximity which brutes would resist'" (7) but which apparently these "classes of people" actually seek out.

Sutherland's confusion reflects the commitment to possessive individualism that disabled structural economic critique. Yet, at the same time, if individuals chose to consume this housing, the notion of the liberal subject that depended on a "natural" desire for the good, including better housing, was at risk. The solution was to assume that these unnatural desires were fostered by the same bad environment that bred disease; the disintegration of the social body would be cured by a medical intervention in the built environment that would in turn act as a kind of medical intervention on the tenants themselves. The incongruity between the model of a sick desire that created and sought a sick environment and an environmentally deterministic model that subsumed the agency of the tenants somehow escaped the attention of sanitary theorists.

By the 1850s, then, the social problems of hygiene were no longer defined solely in terms of nuisance removal; they involved also the people who lived in "problem" environments. Moral health and physical health cannot be separated in this era: in the 1830s it was thought that cholera struck populations that were immoral and excessive in their habits, and by the 1850s it was still largely believed that unsanitary environments resulted as much as, if not more than, from the habits of those who lived within them as from infrastructure or economics. By the 1860s the moral problems of citizenship and inclusion in the social body are understood as involving hygienic self-discipline of individual bodies through moral education, which in turn was dependent upon an environment that would promote moral and cleanly habits. The housing movement itself, although legislatively concerned with sanitation—the destruction of slums, the repair of drains, the construction of new housing up to a certain code—was just as concerned at the level of intervention with the inculcation of domesticity and the performance of privacy, particularly among the lower working classes.

Separating Bodies: Habitus and Desire

In the housing movement, social operations took two peculiar forms. The first was the insistence on the multiplication of rooms for poor families. The second, borrowed directly from the sanitary movement's methods of disease/nuisance control, was house-to-house visitation in order to inculcate appropriate habits. The insistence on multiple rooms peaked in the 1850s and early 1860s. As philanthropic efforts shifted, however, from the artisan to the very poor casual laborer, the emphasis on multiple rooms began to be challenged, especially in 1866–67 by the highly regarded architect Robert Kerr. Although most historians attribute this opposition to a newly realistic attitude toward expenditure, I would argue that it might also be related to the understanding, clearly articulated in the debates surrounding the Second Reform Bill, that residents at this level were not eligible for citizenship, nor would they be eligible until they had acquired not only the physical surroundings but also the desires and habits associated with domesticity as practiced in multiple rooms, practices that privileged privacy, individualism, and bourgeois consumption patterns. Without these desires and habits, multiple rooms were useless. These desires, it was believed, would lead to the economic success required to participate fully in society with an understanding of the differences between public participation and the cultivation of a private self. I would like to focus here on the efforts to inculcate desire for separate rooms and reinforce the distinction between public space and private space in the domestic practices of the poor. I will also discuss Octavia Hill's model of intervention—which became the dominant model for social work—and its use of a maternalist ideal to situate its cultural authority. Hill carefully negotiated between the social and the public, between the need to centralize authority and fit into governmental structures and the need for the social worker to maintain autonomous and private status.

The early nineteenth century saw the creation of suburbs and the middle-class country house and, in urban space, the emergence of architecture reflecting an ever more carefully differentiated culture of privacy. Historian of housing M. J. Daunton summarizes overall changes in architecture and the practice of urban space as follows: "First, the private domain of the house moved from a *promiscuous* sharing of facilities to an *encapsulated* or self-contained residential style. Secondly, the public domain of the city lost a *cellular* quality which had entailed an ambiguous semi-public and semi-private use of space, and took on a much more *open* texture." As a result of this, he argues, dwelling places became more private, and external space, such as doorways and halls, became "totally public, and hence open to view and regulation" (12, his emphasis). Daunton is describing general trends; obviously, working-class housing lagged behind that of the middle classes. Slum clearance and building laws focused on the abolition of courts and dead ends, which over the mid-century abolished the communal, semiprivate space of the court in favor of the wholly public space of the street. When this outdoor space was replaced, it was with individually enclosed yards (24–25). In tenements, however, as Daunton points out, "The threshold between the public and private domain was located in a different manner. . . . The street door led from the public domain into the shared or collective space of the communal stair which was a sort of internal vertical court [elsewhere called the 'upright street']. . . . the lack of privacy . . . had obvious consequences." These consequences were negative for both occupants and landlords (33–34).

Of course, shared sculleries and so forth also contributed to this communality and its discontents, but the stairs seemed to be a more heterogeneous space, less gendered. Many reports cite children playing on the stairs, women or men loitering, talking and drinking there—indeed, very much like the court or street. Daunton also cites the tendency, increasing toward the end of the century, of elites to insist on public space as "waste" space, not to be loitered in. Within private spaces, increased distance between bodies and segregation of rooms became a key concern. The most private of these spaces were those places wherein intimate physical processes were to be secluded from view. Certainly, reformers were concerned about the exposure of children and young adults to sexuality. But, in the words of Edward Gotto, whose concerns were broader, the privy made claims both moral and sanitary: "It is worthy of remark, that this common use of necessaries and water supply has given the place a sort of public character, so that the house, passages, and yards are open all the day, and are the resort of children and idlers, and therefore the inhabitants appear to entertain no idea of privacy." Sanitary improvement, Gotto argued, would restore "domestic comfort" by eliminating "the necessity of making public thoroughfares of private passages, &c." (7–8).

M. J. Daunton notes a number of circumstances converging to contribute to the encapsulation of the working-class home, but he also seems to see it as something of a spontaneous reaction, a natural turning to the family by a working class whose earning and spending power continued to climb throughout the last four decades of the century: "The working class turned away from dependence in their experience of work, toward a search for purpose in the life of the family and home" (266). Certainly, working-class people practiced domesticity in many ways, often oppositional, in this period, and their real physical conditions in terms of health were vastly improved in this period overall. However, Daunton seems to ignore the fact that it was precisely this culture of domesticity, practiced with whatever oppositional autonomy, that in part created the dependence of the working classes on their particular place of work, especially the practice of buying expensive furniture on credit. He also ignores the vocal and concerted efforts of middle-class reformers, builders, and legislators to inculcate this "spontaneously arising" ethic. In addition, he notes the opposition of the working classes to the regulation of public space, and the police's opposition to public sports, gambling, drinking, and so on (266–67), although he credits that resistance to a certain, apparently regressive, segment of the working-class population. It is worth pointing out, though, that the elimination of these shared communal spaces and the practices that went with them necessitated the use of more rooms within the dwelling and more personal possessions to fill them.[1]

Architects interested in the housing problem prioritized privacy as an essential component. Henry Roberts catalogs the components of what he considers a successful project: "The Committee . . . built . . . a 'Model Lodging House' for 104 working men, in which it has been their aim to combine everything deemed essential or valuable . . . complete ventilation and drainage; the use of a distinct living-room; a kitchen and a wash house, a bath, and an ample supply of water; separation and retirement in the sleeping apartments." These and other features were necessary not only for "physical

1. Interestingly, Hill, toward the 1880s and 1890s, when this attack on the use of public space was most strident, recognized the inadequacy of the spaces her tenants had for the practices she wished to inculcate. Yet she acknowledged the value of some kind of communal space and turned not to the street or stairs but to organized group activities such as sewing circles and to the common land movement. Hill was a proponent of the use of graveyards and other small urban greenspaces as local parks for poor tenants. Instead of a liminal or ambiguous border space between public and private (the doorway, the stoop, the stairs), she favors a strict delimitation of private home space and public greenspace, with clearly delineated practices for each, discouraging spontaneous grouping.

comfort" and health but also "to increase their [tenants'] self-respect, and elevate them in the scale of moral and intellectual beings" (9). This project's success is ultimately proved when the tenants weather a bad cholera epidemic with far less mortality than in surrounding buildings.

In Roberts's own proposals, he regrets that separate cottage dwellings are not economically feasible; it will have to be tenements. His concern, therefore, is to make the tenements as separate as possible and to eradicate any communal spaces. Instead of the "vertical court" that indoor stairs tended to become, Roberts suggests, external access to upper-story apartments should be provided by a "gallery carried along the back. . . . This arrangement would obviate many of the evils to be apprehended from internal staircases common to several families" (7).[2] The exterior gallery stairway, he contends, is the best compromise. As far as internal arrangements, separate sleeping rooms (generally intended to be assigned to the parents, the female children, and the male children), "in conformity with the principle of separating the sexes, so essential to decency and morality, are generally three in number, each having its distinct access" (21). There are many such examples.

Those in the housing movement, believing that character is created in the home, argued that housing reform should have priority over educational reform in preparing potential citizens. Housing activists cited teachers' complaints that education could not take place when children arrived dirty, poorly fed, and requiring delousing on an almost daily basis. George Godwin, the influential editor of *The Builder,* the major architectural journal sympathetic to the housing movement, insisted, "Education is but of little use to those living in filthy lanes and such overcrowded dwellings" (*London Shadows* 73). Public support for the housing movement was mobilized by the urban ethnographic literature following Mayhew, which often figured the poor as savages and slums in colonial terms. This literature moves in two directions at once: it positions the poor as Other (savages, from foreign lands) and as Self (disease in the social body, corruption in the heart of the metropole). It also moves in the two directions of realist fiction in this period: it creates and takes advantage of large categories and stereotypes to authenticate its claims (i.e., the particular slum being described is representative of a larger social problem), yet its mobilization of sympathy depends on the literary device of

2. He explains, however, "Some thought it the best adapted and most economical plan to provide in one house, with a common staircase and internal passages, sufficient rooms for lodging a considerable number of families, giving them the use of a kitchen, wash-house and other necessary conveniences, in common; others objected that such an arrangement would lead to endless contentions, and be attended with much evil in cases of contagious disease" (10). Note the linkage of disease and communality.

rendering situations in individual terms. Although the narrator remains an observer—perhaps asking a few questions but rarely otherwise becoming personally involved in the lives of the poor—the move toward individualization and the creation of sympathy places the writings on the feminized, literary side of the social. Godwin wrote many such appeals for public sympathy.

Along with the usual sanitary report–style catalog of horrors, repeatedly related to the cholera epidemics, Godwin insists that any educative or clerical intervention is superfluous until the basic requirements of adequate housing are met. He consistently relates issues of physical hygiene to moral well-being: "Dirty, dilapidated and unwholesome dwellings destroy orderly and decent habits, degrade the character, and conduce to immorality. Bad air produces feelings of exhaustion and lowness of spirits, and these tempt to the use of stimulants—the fruitful parents of all crime" (*London Shadows* 45).[3] He cites sanitary advocates Southwood Smith and also Edwin Bickersteth, best known for his health articles in middle-class journals, to make his point that "the sty makes the pig, not the pig the sty," in opposition to the traditional argument that such places are filthy because of the habits of the people who choose to live there: "'The physical improvement of these masses, it is now admitted, must precede their moral and intellectual elevation'" (Southwood Smith, quoted in Godwin, *London Shadows* 73).[4] This continues the traditional split begun in Chadwick's 1842 report, in which he is at pains both to show that low wages and poverty are *not* the cause of human misery and disease—rather, poor domestic habits are—and simultaneously to argue that money should be spent on housing because proper domesticity is impossible to practice or to teach unless a certain standard of housing is first met: "No education given appears to have availed against such demoralizing circumstances . . . but the moral improvement[s] of a population, by cleansing, draining, and the improvement of the internal and external conditions of the dwellings . . . are more numerous and decided" (200).

Proper domesticity, for Godwin, prerequires an environment with adequate water and separation of rooms. In the habits of his human objects of

3. "A water barrel which would hold fifty or sixty gallons at the most . . . was the only supply furnished for two houses, which, at the lowest calculation, contained a population of one hundred persons, old and young—this to serve for all purposes of cleanliness and domestic use. In this dim undercroft was also the only convenience provided for the same number of persons:—that and the water in close proximity. The smell was abominable. The owners of such places say,—'People of this sort are naturally dirty, and it is useless to do anything with them.' We would ask in reply,—'How is it possible that good habits can be acquired under such circumstances?'" (Godwin, *Town Swamps* 7). Here we see the notion of a habitus necessary to the development of the citizen, without which "natural" desires for cleanliness cannot emerge.

4. Both Bickersteth and Southwood Smith were medics who worked with John Sutherland under Edwin Chadwick, as part of the first General Board of Health.

narration, however, in counterpoint to the usual sanitary problems of overcrowding, drunkenness, inadequately supervised illness, and the keeping of the dead in rooms with the living, Godwin attends to decoration as evidence of "good domestic practice."[5] Apparently, this demonstrates that the dwellers have not only some money beyond what is needed for rent and food but also a taste for the beautiful that indicates proper socialization (it is not incidental that Hill's first housing effort was partially funded by Ruskin). It also shows the inmates' desire and ability to participate in consumer culture; after a long catalog of sanitary horrors and human despair, Godwin proposes, "Let us in a parenthesis, by way of relief from the unpleasantness of the details we are forced to go into, here refer to the love of 'art' which is often exhibited in the most miserable quarters, in the shape of plaster casts and little prints,—not of a very refined character, it is true, but still agreeable and cheering as evidence of a striving upwards" (*Town Swamps* 18).

This "striving upwards" apes the upper classes, supplying evidence of a salutary desire to be like those socially superior to Godwin's subjects: "The painted parrots and spotted cats, and red-and-blue varnished prints, which not many years ago *decorated* homes of greater pretense, have found a resting place lower down in the social scale" (ibid.). Yet at the same time, despite the fact that these same decorations were only recently found in the homes of "greater pretense," they are "not very refined" or even "barbaric": "Our sketch of an actual chimney piece will serve as a record of some well known barbaric favorites. Art offers itself as a social bridge of no ordinary size and strength" (ibid.). There is an uneasiness here that expresses itself as a critique of taste: it is good that the poor wish to have decorations in their home, which proves a domestic impulse. It is even good that in these matters, they are guided by the taste of their superiors (or by the market, which recycles devalued materials that have recently gone out of fashion and makes them accessible to the poor). Yet we must not mistake this decoration as actually "tasteful." This social bridge connects rich and poor but is not to be actually crossed.

Not surprisingly, the heart of this "striving upwards" is the domestic woman, who makes the difference between simply housing and a "home." As we will see in later chapters discussing Dickens and Oliphant, taste is what

5. The social here obviously intersects with Arnoldian notions of culture; culture, too, was seen as a mode of social operations. Once basic social needs were met (and desires created), such as adequate food, cleanliness, and housing, education should follow. Beyond mere literacy, social workers were increasingly convinced that education should focus on taste—hence, we see Ruskinian lectures on classical architecture to members of mechanics' institutes and the opening of museums to the lower classes (on specially designated days of the week). All of these activities were designed to create and direct desire.

both marks the status of the middle-class woman and offers one of her most important contributions to domesticity. Despite hunger and illness in one household, Godwin assures us, "This is not an example of the direst stage of London poverty. . . . There the neat hand of a woman—the world's blessing, and who in her lowest degradation has a perception of the beautiful,—has given a dash of taste to the arrangement" (*London Shadows* 6). Again, it is not simply in its cleanliness but in the decoration of the home that Godwin finds this hopeful quality: "Above the fireplace are several little framed prints [of couples, including the royal family] . . . and a row of small beads are festooned in the centre. On the mantelpiece are various little baskets . . . and other nicknacks of no great value. . . . Poor as this place is, it is still a *home*" (ibid.). Interestingly, what is highlighted in Godwin's description, only partially reproduced here, are detailed descriptions of the prints, which all involved couple and family scenes, culminating in the "young royal family." These, it is presumed, both show a commitment to proper domestic values and demonstrate those values through decoration; the housewife personalizes her home and displays her domesticity through images of other domestic identities with which she claims solidarity, right up to and including the iconic royal family. Her individuality is displayed and her status as a "private" person is enacted through her exercise of taste. She affirms her common humanity through her collection and display of cheap, mass-produced prints, and she proves her domestic values by her reluctance to part with them (she has not sold or pawned them yet). Godwin goes on to muse sadly about the family's probable downward economic trajectory, which will necessitate the sale of these objects; this is, however, too upsetting to contemplate, and so he moves on, he says, to spare the readers' feelings.

The theme of overcrowding, which had become important in the 1840s, was central in the reform literature of the 1860s. It was one of the knottiest problems for legislators. In 1866 MP Mr. Bruce warned, "The House had already dealt with two great causes of disease . . . [water and drainage of nuisances]. But the source of evil the most difficult of all . . . was the overcrowding of houses. . . . In every large town thousands of persons were brought up in a state of moral degradation, which could only end in a great national danger" ("Public Health Bill," 7–8). Individuality could not develop when the people were massed together as contiguous bodies. Chadwick's foundational 1842 "Report on the Labouring Population" devotes a long section to the want of separate apartments.

As described earlier, medical science had also begun to insist on the importance of clean air and the dangerous nature of air "vitiated" by previous breathing. Many doctors determined the healthiness of a building primarily in terms of the number of cubic feet of air per person (ideally 700). However, an underlying concern about "overcrowding" was not the amount of space but its uses. Rodger points out, "It was not simply the physical structures themselves which undermined decency and the family unit—there were many examples of generously proportioned and well maintained terrace housing and tenement flats—it was the congestion with which they were associated" (40–41). Descriptions of persons huddled together in one room usually implicitly, and often explicitly, define incest as an inevitable result of such crowding.[6] "'Talk of morality!'" says sanitarian Edward Bickersteth, in a lecture quoted by Godwin, "'amongst people who herd—men, women, and children—together, with no regard of age or sex, in one narrow, confined apartment! You might as well talk of cleanliness in a sty, or of limpid purity in the contents of a cesspool. . . . The first token of moral life is an attempt to migrate, as though by instinct of self-preservation, to some purer scene'" (in *Town Swamps* 21).

The Three-Room Dogma

The model housing built in the 1840s and 1850s all featured the priority given to multiple rooms, and many reformers were horrified when, despite the availability of a second room, the poor preferred to "pig together" in one room. One sanitary observer disgustedly repudiated one tenant's explanation—that he could not afford to heat another room and the family slept together for warmth—as nonsense; the poor were simply dirty and shameless. Certainly, it is probable that many poor people could not afford second rooms, and when they had them, they could not heat or light them. However, it is also quite possible that many, accustomed to a way of life in which little waking time was actually spent confined to that room, and accustomed to different standards of physical distance, really did find the multiroom lodging oppressive—unnecessary, uncomfortable, and difficult to maintain. In housing the very poor, economic necessity dictated less space, especially in the face of the dictum that there should be no subsidizing to "pauperize" tenants, and the demand for a 5 percent return on investment. Before the mid-1850s, no one had seriously attempted to house the very poor, and so this conflict could be, to some extent, ignored. And despite the fact that most poor people lived in one-room tenements—Daunton cites an 1854 report on cholera in Newcastle that places the proportion of householders in overcrowded single rooms

6. For one out of many examples of an explicit reference to incest, see Chadwick (93).

at approximately half (16)—suggestions that the poor should be offered or encouraged to take single rooms generated storms of controversy. Charles Gatliff argued as early as 1854 that working families did not generally need or use three rooms, but he was unheeded (in Tarn 11)—and even he insisted on separate sculleries and lavatories for each tenement. Robert Kerr's 1866 proposal to provide one-room tenement housing was met with incredulity, despite the fact that he was only suggesting it for households without children at home or headed by single women.

Anticipating some resistance, Kerr begins his argument cautiously: "The suggestion I make in the words *Single room accommodation* may be somewhat startling at first sight; it may well appear strange for an architect to stand here and propose that English families should be confined to the system of single rooms." He urges a scientific attitude to counter the knee-jerk reaction he expects: "those accustomed to professional enquiry will not adopt that precise conclusion until they have heard me further"; then he bases his plea in terms of what the poor really want (and what their finances will bear), rather than what is good for them in the abstract:

> What is it then that the poor really do ask for? The rent, they say, must not be above 4s. per week. This must include taxes and water supply. Then the accommodation must not be too large. . . . It is quite as impossible for a poor man to furnish three or four desirable rooms at a cost of 10L as it is for a poor gentleman to furnish a desirable country house at L5000. Secondly, the accommodation must not be too large for the means of cleaning. . . . And thirdly, the accommodation must not be too complex for the habits of the poor; for their habits are simple and their usage of a house is very rough. . . . Let us ask the labouring man to point us to something which, imperfectly perhaps, but distinctively, indicates or expresses what it is he requires. . . . He points at once to the single room which he has always been accustomed to; it is in fact an institution with him,—improve it as much as you can, but why ignore it?[7] (41)

Not only does Kerr point to the desires of the poor as being as authoritative as economic constraints—an implicit rebuke to philanthropic paternalism (or maternalism), he also argues, against all liberal assumptions of the essential similarity of human desire, that this class of tenants is different in kind from

7. Kerr was an expert on the cost of a large country house, having authored the influential *Gentleman's House* (1864), which recommends a lavish and intricate system of carefully graduated privacies, including separate stairs for men and women.

those who desire two rooms or more. He asks his hearers, "Please to observe there is a radical distinction indicated between these two classes. . . . To live in two rooms is quite a different state of things from living in one room; and this is where I consider the distinction is clearly constituted between the superior labouring class and the inferior labouring class, indicating of course a like distinction as regards the wants of those two classes respectively" (39).

Interestingly, his point—that the people living in one-room dwellings were radically different from those artisans able to afford multiple rooms and should be treated differently— was seen as shockingly regressive, although it would have been a matter of course in the 1830s. Yet his proposal was in some ways perfectly reasonable and, within the constraints of "make it pay" theories of the day, even humane. What particularly jarred the sensibility of his critics was the assumption that the economic distinction indicates "a like distinction as regards the wants" of the classes. That difference, one critic pointed out acidly, if it existed at all, was exactly what they should be trying to correct: "Mr T. Chatfield Clark thought . . . it was a fallacy to say that because the poor were, as a rule, fond of living in one room, persons trying to improve the condition of their dwelling ought not to provide more accommodation." Furthermore, he argued, the poor really did desire at least two rooms: "Those who were acquainted with the habits of the poor . . . would find that there was a strong feeling on the part of right-minded mothers against bringing up a family of children in only one room. What they had to do was to try and give the poor a higher idea of what their condition ought to be" ("Discussion" 50).

So poor people were not fond of living in one room, and if they were, it was because they were not "right minded"; it was the responsibility of the reformer not to indulge them. This is a radical shift from earlier attitudes about the poor, which stressed that they should be encouraged to have quite different wants from the classes above them, according to their station. In the 1860s the emphasis was on the "natural" similarity of the desires of the lower classes to those of the middle and upper classes; if there was a concern about class envy, it was that classes should desire only so much as to make them work to achieve their desires, but not so much as to want to steal or revolt. It is here we see the social at work, leveling difference in the service of the economic. Kerr, in his attitude toward housing the poor, represents an earlier sensibility, although, as Chase and Levenson point out, some of the outrage his proposal generated was surely due to its contradiction of his own obsession with privacy, made the gold standard for the evaluation of housing in his 1864 book, *The Gentleman's House* (174).

Kerr responded to his critics: "some gentlemen . . . seem to think that because I have used the term 'single-room' accommodation, I am to be reproached as a person desirous of perpetuating a debased state of society,—a state of society elegantly described in print as 'pigging together in one room!'" ("Discussion" 62). Exasperated, Kerr calls for the end of the "dogma of the three bedrooms": "When I used the expression 'dogma' . . . I did so advisedly; I meant to signify that it held the position of an accepted doctrine, a credo, not to be any more debated, but to be acted up to as best might be" (76). Undaunted, he sums up his argument thus: "Let us provide . . . above all, some sort of spacious, comprehensive, divisible, single room tenement, as the ordinary standard. . . . The error of all high standards of accommodation has been proved and admitted; but the expediency of keeping to the very lowest standard is not so thoroughly acknowledged" (80). Yet England was moving in the opposite direction—toward a model of citizenship in which the individual's desire for at least two rooms was considered natural, and therefore any model of social intervention that did not posit such an arrangement as necessary was held to be fostering perversion. It is, once again, the management of desire—and desire very specifically directed toward the domestic environment—that will create the conditions for fitness to participate in the life of the nation. In the next chapter we shall take as a case study Octavia Hill's work, which made the management of desire an explicit goal of her housing work.

6

OCTAVIA HILL

Housing as Social Work

> Mere intercourse between rich and poor, if we can secure it without corrupting gifts, would civilise the poor more than anything.
>
> —Octavia Hill, *Our Common Land*

> Beneficence and kindness . . . are relative to a social system which creates the necessity for them by its own inherent defects. Benevolence is beautiful, but it is not based on justice, nor is the "Lady Bountiful" the last word of progress in ethics and civilization.
>
> —L. T. Hobhouse, *Liberalism and Other Writings*

Octavia Hill's Comprehensive Management

In 1866 even Kerr's proposal of room partitioning as a way of producing privacy had not been sufficient to quell the indignation of his critics. By the late 1870s Octavia Hill was still fighting the same battle with a difference; although she believed in the necessity of multiple rooms, pragmatism, she believed, dictated that reformers begin with single rooms and then foster desire for more space. In 1883 she wrote, "Good sized single rooms should be built. . . . Thousands of small poor families . . . want only one large room, . . . indeed prefer it to two small ones. . . . I speak from experience when I say that I know numbers of the prettiest, happiest little homes, which consist of a single room." She adds, "Near to these single rooms, but separable from them, smaller ones should be built which could be let with them, whenever wages, or the standard of comfort, rose. There are many tenants who can be induced by a little gentle pressure and encouragement to spend a rather larger proportion than they now do in rent" (*Homes* 15).

Octavia Hill was one of the earliest social workers, as we now understand the term, who made housing her cause. Her contribution to the improved well-being of hundreds, if not thousands, of Londoners is well documented. She is among the most admirable examples of a Victorian tradition of devotion to social improvement. In this chapter I will be focusing primarily on her to some extent inevitable complicity with bourgeois ideologies, a complicity that is most interesting because it highlights the contradictions of a moment in which Victorian investments in the social were shifting under the weight of its importance to government. But I also want to make clear that this investigation is not denunciatory. It is in understanding the investments of a bourgeois vision of health, domesticity, and the body that we may begin to trace some of the contradictions of a public/private division that we have inherited and with which we continue to struggle.

Octavia Hill provided cheap housing for workers in the city but made housing itself only a part of a comprehensive program of intervention. Hill recognized that her tenants did not necessarily come to her with the desire for the kind of housing that seemed natural to her middle-class colleagues. She believed, however, that it was her duty to inculcate this desire by slow degrees, so that her tenants could eventually internalize her standards and thus reach their natural potential. In this, Hill followed the best wisdom of her political counterparts: first one must create the desire through education; the habits—and the habitus—will follow. In Hill's work and in her negotiation of the boundary between private philanthropy and professional social work, we can see the stratification of the social in action.

Hill never ordered her tenants to do anything other than pay the rent on time. Her goal was to "befriend and persuade," using her considerable cultural and moral authority (backed, not incidentally, by her status as landlady) to mobilize consent. In this way Hill is perhaps the most perfect exemplar of the social; the coercion at the back of social practices is rarely seen as coercion because those practices are seen as the result of natural desire—even if bad environment has so thwarted nature that it requires a little coaxing to reappear. Hill rather proudly relates an instance of "gentle pressure and encouragement":

> They [her tenants] are easily governed by firmness, which they respect much. I have always made a point of carefully recognizing their own rights; but if a strong conviction is clearly expressed, they readily adopt it. . . . One tenant—a silent, strong, uncringing woman, living with her seven children and her husband in one room—was certain "there were many things she could get for the children to eat that would do them more good than another room." I was perfectly silent. A half-pleading, half-asserting voice said: "Don't you see I'm right, miss?" "No," I said; "indeed I do not. I have been brought up to

> know the value of abundant good air; but of course you must do as you think best—only I am sorry." Not a word more passed; but in a few weeks a second room was again to let, and the woman volunteered: "She thought she'd better strive to get the rent; good air was very important, wasn't it?" (*Homes* 21)

We can easily see why Beatrice Webb and Henrietta Barnett criticized Hill for her arrogance and "hypocritical" cordiality to the poor (Boyd 134); from a present-day perspective the emphasis on space over food seems particularly inhumane. Such rhetoric is easily satirized, and indeed, in a later chapter, we will see what an accomplished comic writer such as Margaret Oliphant can do with such promising material, in her humorlessly managerial "stateswoman" Miss Marjoribanks. But Hill did not differ signally from other housing reformers on this point; what was different about her approach was the personalized relationship she insisted on with her tenants and—paradoxically—the amount of "freedom" the tenants had to make their own decisions. While it is easy in retrospect to identify the inconsistencies of Victorian liberal positions, it is, of course, also important to emphasize that, within existing value systems and knowledges, activists such as Hill were progressive and made real differences for the better in many people's lives, which is not a negligible achievement. I will focus here on the problems rather than the achievements of Victorian liberalisms in part because those problems remain acute today, and this kind of genealogical analysis can best trace the origins and effects of the assumptions we still carry within our own vision of social work.

Managing Space

Hill's general policy on space also reflects her understanding of both the economic aspects of her tenants' lives and the fact that the real target of social management is the desires of the poor, rather than practices that will quickly be abandoned as soon as surveillance can no longer be maintained: "With the great want of room in this neighborhood, it did not seem right to expel families, however large, inhabiting one room. Whenever . . . a room was vacant, and a large family occupied an adjoining one, I have endeavored to induce them to rent the two. . . . At first they considered it quite an unnecessary expenditure . . . [but] . . . they have gradually learnt to feel the comfort of having two rooms, and pay willingly for them" (*Homes* 22). It was believed that housing had to pay at least 5 percent on investment and to be affordable to the poor without subsidy, in order both to be economically viable on a wide scale and to avoid pauperizing the tenants, which would counter the whole purpose of socialization that housing was to provide. Somehow this had to be accomplished in high-cost urban areas, owing to the necessity for the poor to be close to employment. Anthony Ashley Cooper, the Earl of Shaftesbury's and others' model lodging schemes targeted the poor artisan but left untouched the population of the lower working class on the verge of pauperism, but this was precisely the class targeted for intervention under the pressures of the late 1850s and 1860s, as England moved toward its second reform. A model for modern social work, Octavia Hill's project included not only housing the very poor but also intimately managing and counseling them. Her work dramatizes the operation of the social, its opportunities for middle-class women, and also the limits of those opportunities.

Managing Desire

With all the room imaginable, it still could not be guaranteed that the tenants would use it correctly. Therefore, the key to social and sanitary reform was house-to-house visitation. This practice evolved as a form of observation in the campaign to control epidemics; only by seeing the interiors of households and their occupants could the observer determine the salubrity of the surroundings or the morbidity of the dwellers. Intervention initially took the form of forced clearance of nuisances and removal of the sick and dead; later, it came in dispensing tickets for medicine and mandating the removal of persons not in the immediate family in cases of overcrowding. Friendly or philanthropic visiting, the other form of house-to-house visitation, saw itself as tutelage by example—as Hill put it, "living side by side with people, til all that one believes becomes clear to them" (in Lewis 6–7).

Philanthropic visiting was often imagined nostalgically in terms of a lady-of-the-manor relationship with the poor (as in Ruskin's *Of Queen's Gardens*); Hill in particular envisions herself as creating a kind of community within the faceless overcrowding of the urban center, a community she believes existed before industrialization. As landlady, of course, she had particular claims to that analogy. Hill, however, did not merely see herself, as so many before her did, as establishing a particular and small community of support for some poor. She saw herself as "governing" the desires of the poor in their own interest and as teaching those who were outside of the social body to behave in a manner that might bring them within it.[1] The language with which

1. In France, this role is made explicit much earlier: as early as 1820, in Joseph-Marie de Gerando's manual for visitors of the poor, the philanthropist is admonished to investigate the lives of

visiting is described generally in this period reflects the missionary nature of the project; Godwin asserts that "To investigate the condition of the houses of the very poor in this great metropolis is a task of no small danger and difficulty: it is necessary to brave the risks of fever and other injuries to health, and the contact of men and women often as lawless as the Arab or the Kaffir" (*London Shadows* 1).

Hill, however, although vitally interested in improving physical environment, insisted on the reciprocal relationship between teaching adequate habits and providing adequate homes, at least beyond a certain minimal level of cleanliness and structural integrity:

> That the spiritual elevation of a large class depended to a considerable extent on sanitary reform was, I considered, proved; but I was equally certain that sanitary improvement itself depended upon education work among grown-up people; that they must be urged to rouse themselves from the lethargy and indolent habits into which they have fallen, and freed from all that hinders them from doing so. I further believed that any lady who would help them to obtain things, the need of which they felt themselves, and would sympathize with them in their desire for such, would soon find them eager to learn her view of what was best for them; that whether this was so or not, her duty was to keep alive their own best hopes and intentions . . . governing more than . . . helping.[2] (*Homes* [1866] 17–18)

She reflects, "Mere intercourse between rich and poor, if we can secure it without corrupting gifts, would civilise the poor more than anything" (*Our Common Land* 98).

The visitor's authority depends on two things equally: her status as a lady and her sympathy with their needs. On the one hand, she is a social and economic authority figure (and exerts direct authority as landlady, in Hill's case); on the other, she is a private individual, in a relationship of equality and what Poovey would call "structural equivalence." It is particularly important that it be a "lady," not a "gentleman"—the lady's moral authority is based in the private and the social, on her domestic identity. The striking thing in reading Hill is not her casual assertion of the authority of her position as "governor"

---

the recipients closely. "*Morality was systematically linked to the economic factor*, involving a continuous surveillance of the family" (Donzelot 69, his emphasis).

2. Although Hill's writings were gathered into books, they were first published as essays. When I cite Hill's writings in this chapter, I include the dates of first publication in brackets. The page numbers, however, are from the books in which the essays were collected and reprinted; these sources are in the Works Cited

of her tenants, which is frequently present, but her equally frequent insistence on her relationship as friend and equal—her denial that she exerts any authority save that of reason and example. In her insistence on a government by consent, which masks any reference to her power, and on the separation of the private (her friendships) from the economic (Hill was unyielding in her rule that anyone who did not pay rent on time would be turned out), and finally in her belief that the separation of the economic from the private was mutually supportive with her moral goals for tenants' behavior, Hill embodies the precise contradictions and ideals of liberal government in the period.

Managing Individuals

Hill's method depended on relations of intimacy with her tenants: "My people are numbered, not merely counted, but known, man, woman, and child. . . . Think of what this mere fact of *being known* is to the poor!" (*Homes* [1869] 34–35). The choice of words here, I think, is particularly opportune. The investigative side of the social is the side that "counts" the poor, abstracting them into specific information; Hill's method does not oppose this but rather supplements it—the poor who are counted by sanitary authorities are "numbered" by her in the biblical sense. There is a practical aspect, of course: being "known" means that the very poor have some access to the cultural capital of a higher economic class—they can get references for jobs and take advantage of some of the tutelary networking available to more skilled and long-term laborers. But more to the point, being known as individuals by someone who "matters" demassifies the poor person as an unreasoning atom of a large unreasoning mass and reconstructs that person in the image of bourgeois individualism—there is someone there with a unique and valuable subjectivity to "know."

Hill also means that she can "know" them because they are not the Other—their desires are "known" because they are similar to hers as part of the same social body. They are structural equivalents with the same goals, because they both belong to families that are "natural" and therefore identical in operation:

> I have heard . . . girls themselves, fevered with desire to do more, talk rather enviously of those who can give their time wholly to such work; but have they ever thought how much is lost by such entire dedication?—or, rather, how much is gained by her who is not only a visitor of the poor, but a member

> of a family with other duties? It is the families, the homes of the poor, that need to be influenced. Is she not the most sympathetic, most powerful, who nursed her own mother through her long illness, and knew how to go quietly about the darkened room; who entered so heartily into the sister's love and marriage; who obeyed so perfectly the father's command when it was hardest? Better still if she be wife and mother herself, and can enter into the responsibilities of a head of a household, understands her joys and cares, knows what heroic patience it needs to keep gentle when the nerves are unhinged and the children noisy. Depend upon it, if we thought of the poor primarily as husbands, wives, sons and daughters, members of households, as we are ourselves, instead of contemplating them as a different class, we should recognize better how the house training and high ideal of home duty was our best preparation for work among them. . . . What, in comparison with these gains is the regularity of the life of the weary worker, whose life tends to make her deal with people en masse, who gains little fresh springs from other thoughts and scenes? For what is it that we look forward to as our people gradually improve? Not surely to dealing with them as a class at all, any more than we should tell ourselves off to labour for the middle classes, or aristocratic class, or shop-keeping class. Our ideal must be to promote the happy mutual intercourse of neighbors. . . . If we establish a system of professed workers, amateur or paid, we shall quickly begin to hug our system, and perhaps to want to perpetuate it even to the extent of making work for it. (*Our Common Land* 24–27)

Several important points can be made about this interesting statement. Hill believes that the moral authority of middle-class women emerges from the similarities of their lives with those of the poor in the universals of sickness, nursing, patriarchal structure, and so on. (Obviously, this elides the differences between homes with servants and adequate food and water and those that have none, or between the expected patriarchal structure and the frequent occurrence of unwed motherhood, to name a few examples.) The statement that the "most sympathetic" is "most powerful" deflects attention from the coercive aspect of power and grounds power in equivalence, which is explicitly counterpoised to class; in fact, the goal of this exercise in sympathy is to erase class, not by improving the person's economic situation, although that may be part of the process, but by erasing the significance of economic difference. But perhaps most interesting of all is Hill's suspiciousness of professional social workers. Despite the fact that Hill did much to create an institutional context and method for social work, and that students of social work came from the Continent and North America to study her method, Hill opposed the professionalization of social work until the end of her life.[3]

Maternalism and Professionalism

Hill's reaction to the style of intervention based on Jane Addams's Hull House, in which a community of women live domestically within the area in which they are working, is that these "Homes" are false—they are not really replicative of patriarchal nuclear families, and worse, they make work with the poor central, rather than an extension of home duties. Too close to professionalism, they were also not "real" homes: "Much has been written of late on the subject of Sisterhoods and of 'Homes' . . . I must here express my conviction that we want very much more the influence that emanates not from a 'Home,' but from 'homes'" (*Homes* 66). She wanted her visitors to relate to the poor as neighbors, not as professionals or missionaries: "I hope for a return of the old fellowship between rich and poor . . . to men and women coming out from bright, good, simple homes, to see, teach, and learn from the poor; returning to gather fresh strength from home warmth and love, and seeing in their own homes something of the spirit which should pervade all" (*Homes* 66).[4] Such an attitude of distrust of professional social workers was widespread in the 1860s, and such workers are perhaps most famously lampooned in Dickens's *Bleak House,* in which Mrs. Jellyby and Mrs. Pardiggle's own families are miserable and neglected in favor of the ladies' pet causes, which are never really advanced by the philanthropists' efforts.[5] In contrast, Dickens offers us the unpretentious but effective help of Esther, who simply reaches out from within her own family, letting her "circle of duty" expand to include those

3. Nancy Boyd remarks of Hill's system, "The ideal manager combines two principles: she is to participate as 'a volunteer,' that is 'a spontaneous undertaker of tasks' . . . and she is to be trained as a 'professional,' a worker whose knowledge of science, sociology and economics enables her to reconcile the care of individual tenants with the needs of the community. . . . In later life, Octavia Hill expressed reservations about the . . . increasing tendency of workers to specialize. . . .The professional status of the visitors might be considered to make them superior to their clients, yet as volunteers they can be equals" (153–54).

4. Dorice Williams Elliott argues in another context that Octavia Hill can be called a "professional philanthropist" because she did philanthropy "full time," believed in rigorous training, and came to be a publicly recognized "expert" (204). Certainly, as she observes, this introduced a new level of rigor and commitment—and standardization—to the practice. However, as we have seen, Hill herself would have considered this more a matter of following one's avocation with a proper regard for its success than as a profession per se.

5. Seth Koven's *Slumming* also offers an excellent reading of the narratives of sexual impropriety and same-sex desire associated with women philanthropists in this period.

whose lives she can personally touch and improve. (Of course, other novelists' lady philanthropists were more heroic: witness Rhoda Broughton's Kate in *Not Wisely but Too Well* (1867), who becomes a Sister of Mercy, or Mary Ward's pauper-nurse in the 1894 novel *Marcella.*)

Despite her desire that visitors should not professionalize, Hill worked hard to establish relationships between visitors and bodies such as the Poor Law Commissioners. Her proposal was twofold: a method for visitors to follow and a centralized structure of authority. Firmly believing, as many Victorians did, that charity was often pauperizing and that too often aid was dispensed in ways that harmed recipients rather than helped them to achieve independence, Hill believed that all charities should work together through a centralized agency, the COS (Charities Organization Society) and, in turn, with institutional bodies like the Poor Law Commissioners, to coordinate aid and, most crucially, share information so that recipients of aid could be properly tracked and managed in light of their personal histories. She proposed an elaborate system of organization involving the visitors, whose job it was to know the poor thoroughly and decide when and what kind of help should be given or withheld, and an intermediary female supervisor who would have some knowledge of the Poor Law and the workings of government. The visitors would report to the supervisors and take direction from them; in turn, the supervisors would report to the male administrators of local church and government bodies, as well as charity boards of various descriptions.

The advantages of this system were, she argued, that a more accurate sense of needs could be determined, since the poor were unreliable and inarticulate about their own needs; that follow-up could be performed within the context of the "friendship" of the visitor; and that all efforts could be brought to bear in terms of including the poor within the social body rather than providing short-term melioration (sometimes this might even involve forcing someone into the workhouse rather than helping her to manage a little longer; the sense is that the workhouse is inevitable in some cases, and it is better to institutionalize the hopeless sooner rather than having them loose). Why, then, in this elaborate and highly formalized system, is it important to maintain the "front line" of workers as nonprofessionals? Again, it is based on the notion of sympathy and equivalence: "The Relief Committee . . . have before them not only the valuable information of the Charity Organization Society, . . . but also the detailed account of a volunteer, who brings to bear on the case a fresher and more personal sympathy than a paid agent ordinarily possesses, who has much more patience to listen to, and probably more patience to elicit the little facts upon which so much may depend" (*Homes* 58). Hill's insistence on equality has often been dismissed as disingenuous. However, most observers miss the point of Hill's sense of community with her tenants. It is not that Hill thought of them as social equals; she did not. Her friendship extended to inviting them to her home—in a special room that she built on at the back and that she also used for rent collection. The point was not to achieve social equality with her tenants; it was that she believed them to be potential participants in the social body and public sphere—citizens whose interests (narrowly defined) counted equally with her own.

Citizen and Nation

Hill's sense of her tenants as potential citizens was reflected in her insistence on the oneness of national community. She emphasized both the necessity and the danger of local community: local community is good, and activism should begin in one's own neighborhood because one must conceive of community as a group of individuals with whom one's relationships were personal. But that was valuable only insofar as, like one's own family, it enabled one to sympathetically understand and claim solidarity with other families, other communities. To the extent that it was used as a marker of identity, such as class, it became dangerous. As she exhorted her fellow workers, "Is humanity, is nationality, is citizenship too large for our modern love or charity to embrace, and shall it in future be limited to our family, our successful equals, or our superiors?" (*Our Common Land* 90–91). She saw centralization as part of that process, reflecting that one should feel part of a larger whole than one's "ecclesiastical parish"—and did, thanks to the COS (ibid., 168). One's family, properly conducted, would enable one to enlarge one's sympathies to include other families. Local identities that were not connected to a larger sense of community actually caused community to degenerate. She pressed her colleagues:

> I would urge you all who are inhabitants of a large parish, markedly divided into poor and rich districts, as citizens of a city fearfully so divided, to weigh well your duties; and, never forgetting the near ones to home and neighborhood, to remember also that when Europe is sacrificed to England, England to your own town, your own town to your parish, your parish to your family, the step is easy to sacrifice your family to yourself. (*Our Common Land* 172–73)

Hill saw her "raw" tenants as riven by local identity, citing quarrels between English and Irish women and the lack of a sense of permanence in tenants' dwellings as failing to allow for neighborly bonding. But most of all, an inadequate sense of family responsibilities and relationships kept poor people from having possibilities of sympathy for one another, in Hill's view—community arises out of the sense of structural equivalence that begins with one's identity within a family.[6] Hill took on the role of mother, pleased when her tenants shelved their differences to please her, as, according to her, they often did.

Hill also provided classes at some of her tenements; about bringing women together for classes, sewing, and cleaning, she writes, "a neighborly feeling is called out among the women as they sit together on the same bench, lend one another cotton or needles. . . . The babies are a great bond of union. . . . That a consciousness of corporate life is developed in them is shown by the not infrequent use of the expression 'One of us'" (*Homes* [1869] 28). The neighbors share health information and stories of child development; out of this comes the sense of an "us" that Hill so prizes. What is remarkable about this moment is that Hill utterly fails to note any of the other bonds of community remarked upon by historians of the working classes and that are so evident in the communal uses of stairs, courts, and the like (even the women fighting probably see themselves in a communal relationship of some sort); nor does she regard the common experience of shared labor habits or economic struggle as a legitimate source of communal feeling. Moreover, it is not simply that Hill decries this as a less legitimate source of communal feeling; it is that she does not see it at all. Her triumphant citation of the common phrase "one of us" may indicate that this phrase was rarely used by her tenants; it more likely indicates that it was rarely used in a manner that Hill recognized as meaningful.

Professionalizing Social Work

Finally, of course, the Victorian model of the social as profoundly separate from government could no longer withstand the pressure of its centrality to the aims of government itself, and social work became professionalized—both

6. The belief that permanence was necessary to community feeling can be seen in Mayhew's anxiety about the peripatetic nature of the costermongers. Middle-class residents could not understand how any bond of community could be experienced by workers constantly on the move. Rodger quotes several studies to show that Victorian working-class people moved often; for example, in mid-Victorian Liverpool in 1871, 40 percent moved within one year. However, workers generally moved over short distances, within range of existing family connections. Middle-class residents, whose sense of home was firmly anchored to a particular building, probably had a much more restricted understanding of neighborhood than some working-class residents, who may have seen themselves as "at home" within a space composed of certain urban itineraries rather than a particular address.

the ultimate success and failure of Hill's ideal. Hill was active from the 1860s through the end of the century; she never swerved from her firm commitment to volunteerism and tutelage of the poor. Only in private, individual relationships, paradoxically, could the aims of nation be bodied forth and realized:

> The people's homes are bad, partly because they are badly built and arranged; they are tenfold worse because the tenants' habits and lives are what they are. . . . There needs . . . a reformatory work which will demand the loving zeal of individuals which cannot be had for money, and cannot be legislated for by Parliament. The heart of the English nation will provide it—individual, reverent, firm, and wise. It may and should be organized, but cannot be created. (*Homes* [1883] 10)

Nationhood depends both on individuality and on the sense of community called forth by volunteerism; professionalizing social work would destroy that bond of sympathy between individual private persons upon which both Habermas's public sphere and the social are based, and upon which citizenship and consent are founded. The eradication of *private* characteristics in that work, therefore, would make it ineffective in producing the social. Economic aid can be given by the masculinized professional, but only from a position of privacy can the domestic feminine intervene in and produce the fragile privacy of the newly socialized poor. And only then may the poor emerge into and through the social into the social body itself as bearers of a public, and proudly English, identity.

Hill believed that her highly individualized work, based on the private, feminine concerns of domesticity and family, would have profound reverberations in the public sphere, but she did not believe that work that began there or defined itself thus could "trickle down" in the other direction. Hill was one of the many women activists who concentrated on "social" problems yet contributed profoundly to female visibility in the public sphere and female discussion of issues that came to be defined as "women's issues"—home safety, children's health, and so on—that have been taken up by feminist and other activists today. These women have left legacies, of models for both social work and women's activism. Within these legacies, however, the primacy of the private and individual has continued to pose problems for workers wishing to emphasize the vital connection between structural inequities and individual suffering, just as today, professional social work still favors an individualist casework model, with continued "natural" distinctions in dealing with "criminal" and "family" violence whose effects are often not so easily distinguishable as we presume their contexts to be.

Most social workers in the United States today are female, especially social workers involved with family issues (as opposed to, for example, parole officers). In a volume which instructs home visitors, Hoover and colleagues point out that "the number of programs utilizing [prophylactic] home visiting as a strategy for delivering services has rapidly expanded" in the 1990s (17), and they identify the key goals of home visiting as role modeling and providing "social support" by "developing a trusting relationship" (18). The text admonishes them to "keep the home a home," noting that "home should be where families can retreat from other influences or pressures of the outside world" (51). This rather Victorian distinction between domestic and public sphere not only emphasizes a discontinuity between private and public but also fails to acknowledge that traumatic incidents are very likely to occur within the domestic sphere—indeed, in the case of women and children, more likely to occur within than outside it. In England and Wales the casework model of social work also predominates (Payne 172), despite a tradition of theoretical emphasis among many social workers on structural inequalities (ibid., 178). In the United States the trend has been even more heavily individualist (Leighninger and Midgley 11, 23); although recent discussions have focused on issues of social justice, these almost always translate in practice to an emphasis on avoiding harmful stereotypes and respecting cultural difference in working with individual "clients."

The persistent separation of domestic and public, and the partial persistence of their gender investments, have continued to baffle activists who recognize a clear continuity between the two and yet face an ideological barrier that depoliticizes domestic problems and the social problems that are still seen as continuous with them. Despite exhortations that the personal is political, or the more recent admonishment to think globally, act locally (are those connected by "and" or "but"?), the political is still often not recognized as personal: domestic violence is still a woman's issue and family poverty is still a social—in contrast to an economic or political—issue. Social work, despite a nod to systems-based approaches, enacts that approach in the United States overwhelmingly as psychological intervention, and union activism is still not recognized as social work.

How successful were Hill and her ilk? Historians of housing usually consider this question from the perspective of economics. While some argue that Hill made great strides in proving that housing the poor was economically viable, most see her as regressive, retarding the advent of subsidized housing. Richard Rodger sums up his view of the question: "[It is highly doubtful that] by intervening in the housing market, philanthropy redefined laissez-faire attitudes. . . . Arguably it buttressed existing ideology, superimposing middle-class emphases on private property and repayment of debts upon a working-class preference for communality and neighborliness." He concludes that model housing was finally no more than "a marginal social experiment, delaying radical approaches," though he credits its failure with hastening the acceptance of municipal intervention (46).

Hill's major contribution, however, should be understood not merely within a teleology of housing history that moves toward subsidy as its (now endangered) end, but in the context of the history of the social. Hill is part of a period that elaborates a science of social work that organized philanthropy under the sign of sanitary science and then used its authority to encompass and subordinate public medicine to the larger aims of the social. Her real success was in modeling a way in which those outside the social body could be brought within it, and in making effective bridges between the weak legislation that was available and intervention workers. The partial and contradictory efforts to institute sanitary change—the 1848 Health of Towns Act, the multiple housing acts up to and including Torrens and Cross—were mobilized, used, and made more effective by a large network of social workers.

The institution of domesticity in at least the poorer working classes met with both successes and failures from the social worker's point of view. The incorporation of the working poor into a larger social body tied together by consumer desire for mass-produced items was fairly successful. Ironically, this desire often led to what we might call "level-jumping" in the performance of domestic privacy, which exasperated and mystified middle-class reformers. For example, the desire for a parlor seen among the working classes at the end of the century often led to the use of the "extra" or third room in ways housing reformers had not anticipated. (These homes, which were not occupied by the extremely poor, usually had two bedrooms upstairs and two rooms downstairs, a kitchen and parlor, plus a scullery in the backyard.) Representing respectability and status, the parlor became the home of expensive furniture and pianos purchased on credit, rarely used except for special occasions—thus causing the family to remain crowded in fewer rooms. "The result was a strong emphasis on the distinction between the front and back of the house. . . . There was an often articulated desire [among the residents] to escape from promiscuous mixing and sharing" (Daunton 277). (According to Daunton, this reflects the shift from being work-centered to home-centered among the working classes.)[7] So the desire for a middle-class version of

7. Although middle-class observers saw this practice as a both a foolish expenditure and an underutilization of space, as Daunton observes, it was still not possible for many families at this income to consistently heat two "living rooms," and thus the kitchen became the living room as well as the kitchen, and both cooking and washing were relegated to the scullery (280–81), the everyday

domesticity prioritized public display (the parlor) and family retirement (the move to the back of the house) over the middle-class model of the domestic practice of space by the family that, by middle-class standards, should have preceded and legitimated the relatively superfluous display space of the parlor. However, this choice points out that middle-class respectability and legitimacy were unerringly located by working-class homemakers in the *display* of domestic privacy indicated by the possession of a "buffer" room between public and private, and not within the actual domestic practices hidden (and therefore immaterial, because invisible) within the back rooms of the house. This display became particularly important in marking small differences in neighborhoods largely homogenous in economic status and architecture: "While income gradations between skilled and unskilled, clerks and the middle class existed, similarities within each socioeconomic sub-group, defined by ideals and cultural values, were given greater coherence by virtue of residential proximity" and by small differences in vernacular architecture that proclaimed status (Rodger 28).

Despite the continuation of a "commonsense" model of the social as profoundly separate from government, its centrality to the aims of government could not be ignored. Social work became professionalized and uneasily integrated into the technologies of government. The same unease evoked by the incomplete separation of the social from the political that we see in Hill's work was a topic of interest to mid-century novelists. The social in its relation to the political was a site of both opportunity and danger, especially for women. In the next three chapters, we will see how several novelists addressed this thorny issue.

---

use of the parlor space not being practical. Of course, seasonal changes in expenditures or income often necessitated the taking in of a lodger, which reorganized the use of space yet again.

SECTION III

Narrating the Citizen of the Social

7

THE POLITICAL NOVEL AND THE SOCIAL

> There are people who are very tragical about village nuisances, and there are other people who assail them with loathing . . . but Lucilla [had] . . . the liveliest satisfaction to think of all the disorder and disarray. . . . Her fingers itched to be at it.
>
> —Margaret Oliphant, *Miss Marjoribanks*

> There is a lesson for you fine ladies, who think you can govern the world by what you call your social influences . . . [as] a reward for great exertions, or, if necessary, an inducement to infamous tergiversation.
>
> —Benjamin Disraeli, *Coningsby*

From the 1840s on, a groundswell of novels attempted to mediate between the public and private, the political and the social spheres. Grounding the public in narratives of nation that were sometimes elaborated through racial discourses, they document an uneasy fascination with the relationship of the social to the political. Taking for granted the primacy of a middle-class vision of interiority and individualism, these novels operate not only as powerful arguments in their own right but also as forces that inculcate as truth the assumptions underlying their arguments. Like Octavia Hill's work, these novels are often implicitly politically engaged, operating as arguments for or against social change, and sometimes explicitly supporting particular legislation. As works of art with appeal over a long period of time, however, rather than commentaries self-evidently aimed at addressing a particular historical moment and issue, these novels go much further than, say, parliamentary speeches to normalize the assumptions about the social and the self that underlie them and form their conditions of possibility. Because the novel was largely devoted to narratives of individual development and consciousness, it was a form in which the association between the proper body and mind was inevitably primary. These writers took as their theme the connection of the social and the political, linking that connection to a specific kind of individual (and individualist) body and consciousness required for fitness. The novels also, however, coming decades after the first reform debates, contain some wry critiques of the porousness of the boundaries between domains. Sanitary science and the tutelage of the middle-class woman are key to producing the healthy body of the fit citizen, but women's social power comes dangerously close to political influence, perhaps in part because public opinion is itself feminized.

Sybil, Sanitation, and Social Liberalism

In his 1845 political novel *Sybil,* Disraeli uses race, in the manner made familiar to British readers by Carlyle and other writers, to undergird his narrative of nation. Egremont and Sybil are of the Norman and Saxon race, respectively, and the accession of Victoria is the enthronement of a queen who "has the blood and beauty of the Saxon. Will it be her proud destiny to . . . break the last links in the chain of Saxon thralldom?" (62). That thralldom is, of course, the enslavement of the "People" and the "Sovereign" to nasty imported political notions—a "Venetian Parliament" and a system of "Dutch finance."[1] It is the "Saxon multitudes," according to Disraeli, who make up the group of oppressed laborers, and non-Saxons are represented only by one "good Irishman" who helps Sybil when she is lost in a dangerous slum. The speech of the noble labor leader, Gerard (who is, of course, unbeknownst to himself, actually a Saxon aristocrat), is given at the Druid's Altar (328). Fortunately, Disraeli, the once and future Tory, is there to lead the way "to bring back strength to the Crown, liberty to the Subject, and to announce that power has only one duty: to secure the social welfare of the People" (416).

However, the Saxons are not merely innocent and noble victims; nor are the Normans only exploiters. The Machiavellian labor leader Morley leads the "hell cats"—inhabitants of a village so barbaric that it has no church and is consecrated to Woden—in the riot and burning of a castle in which they themselves, having become drunk on their spoils, are immolated. Egremont comes to see that his mission is the (social, not political) liberation of the people, whereas the "Woden worshippers" who riot in the name of labor are "savages" who die for their presumption—only, however, after destroying the Norman castle of the socially irresponsible Lord Marney. Improbably, the two "good" groups—responsible Normans and civilized Saxons—are reconciled in the marriage of Egremont and Sybil.

1. This theory is more fully described in *Coningsby* (see especially 351–60 and 366–69).

The evils of "enthralled" Saxondom are described extensively in sanitary terms, first of housing, and then of nuisances: "The gaping chinks admitted every blast. . . . Before the doors of these dwellings . . . ran open drains full of animal and vegetable refuse, decomposing into disease" (78). The filth, manure, and resulting diseases are described for several pages. This is a village to which agricultural laborers have been driven as a result of Lord Marney's unwillingness to be responsible for them on his own land. By contrast, Mr. Trafford, the progressive factory owner, "recognised the baronial principle" (277) and builds a village for his workers, knowing "that the domestic virtues are dependent on the existence of a home" (276). Though he was the principal proprietor, he "encouraged his workmen to purchase the fee" (276), fostering individual ownership and upward mobility. This village is a sanitary miracle, with a well in every street and public baths, and the workers are constantly "observed" and "encouraged" (276).

Disraeli manages to take on most of the sanitary and social issues of the day. "Infanticide," he says, "is practiced as extensively and as legally in England as it is on the banks of the Ganges" (146), referring to the practice of working-class English baby minders keeping their charges quiet with opium. Disraeli's character "Devilsdust" (perhaps a gloss on Carlyle's Teufelsdrockh), an otherwise nameless and abandoned working-class child who has somehow survived the ills that carried off all the other children at the baby minder's (146–47), becomes an organic intellectual and advocate of the rights of labor. This character, however, reappears after the riot and fire as a married "capitalist" in a firm that, Disraeli assures us, will eventually "furnish . . . a crop of members of Parliament and Peers of the Realm" (639)—a classic narrative of property conferring fitness, though clearly an exceptional case. In short, though Disraeli highlights the nearly impossible conditions that kill Devilsdust's childhood companions, he finally retains a "self-made" success story in which the most abject of these children teaches himself to read, becomes a radical, then grows into a capitalist himself and drops politics altogether—except, perhaps, to produce new generations who will enter Parliament representing capitalist interests. Meanwhile, the proper class to practice politics is the political class, such as Egremont himself, who will represent Devilsdust and his kin so much more adequately than they could themselves, in their delusional pursuit of suffrage.

Sybil, the Chartist maiden, like Elizabeth Gaskell, comes to attribute "the want of sympathy that unquestionably exists between Wealth and Work in England, to mutual ignorance between the classes which possess those two great elements of national prosperity" (442), rather than economic struggle. Young Englandist Egremont, like Eliot's Felix Holt, advocates the "results of the Charter without the intervention of its machinery" in what is described as a "really democratic speech" (429), wherein he declares that "the social happiness of the millions should be the first object of statesman" (443), and that social happiness is to be procured through sanitary intervention, education, and housing, not political activity. Egremont argues that England's is "the mind ever of the rising race" (447) and that the "future principle of English politics will not be a levelling principle. . . . It will seek to ensure equality, not by levelling the Few, but by elevating the Many" (448). Using, in short, a teleology of racial and social progression as a national master-narrative grounded on the healthy (Saxon) body—that he will in later novels complicate with his ill-received "Eastern" political superhero, Sidonia—Disraeli offers social liberalism with political Toryism, to be achieved through sanitary and social reform.

Unlike many liberals, however, Disraeli has scant sympathy with franchise reform. In *Sybil* of 1845 he charges that the First Reform Bill has linked the mean pursuit of wealth with fitness in a manner antithetical to public-spiritedness:

> If a spirit of rapacious covetousness, desecrating all of the humanities of life, has been the besetting sin of England for the last century and a half, since the passing of the Reform Act the altar of Mammon has blazed with triple worship. To acquire, to accumulate, to plunder each other . . . to propose a Utopia to consist only of WEALTH and TOIL, this has been the breathless business of enfranchised England for the last twelve years. (47)

Although reform also has had some good effects in engaging the public in political thinking, Disraeli warns that it has also created a credulous polis liable to be misled: it has "led the public mind to ponder somewhat on the circumstances of our national history. . . . It created and prepared a popular intelligence to which one can appeal . . . in an attempt to dispel the mysteries with which . . . it has been the labour of party writers to involve a national history" (ibid.). Clearly this is disingenuous: Disraeli appeals to a conspiracy theory in which party leaders, acting up to principles in public that they secretly abjure, have deliberately disseminated a false national history that Disraeli will reveal as a "Venetian" plot. This has resulted in "serfage" for the people. But Disraeli will give us a dazzling new plan, much in the mode of Carlyle, with some Monarchist trappings, and including all the latest accessories from sanitary science. This plan carefully separates politics from the social. Indeed, political interest among the people indexes the breakdown of a proper division between the public and the private: the public pursuit of the social well-being of the people and the private pursuit of wealth and societal preferment have become entangled, at the expense of the legitimate pursuits of public life.

Politics cannot offer a forum for the development of the self or the nation, having degenerated into mere theater because of the damaging influence of public opinion. On the theatrical nature of politics, Disraeli notes that the Chartists failed to distinguish clearly between the two parties: "And they were right. . . . Where is the distinctive principle? A shadowy difference may be simulated in opposition, to serve a cry . . . but the mask is not worn, even in Downing Street; and the conscientious conservative seeks, in the pigeonholes of a whig bureau, for the measures which for ten years he has been sanctioning, by the speaking silence of an approving nod, a general wail of frenzied alarm" (417). Mr. Tadpole, the anxious political advisor, observes that "private character is to be the basis of the new government. Since the Reform Act, that is a qualification much more esteemed by the country than public services" (402). His interlocutor agrees that "this is a domestic country" (401–2), thus affirming that character is a domestic issue, carefully cordoned off from the issue of public or political actions.

It is an ambiguous critique, though, since Disraeli denounces the First Reform Bill, "a mean and selfish revolution which emancipated neither Crown nor People" (641), as empty theater, and since the person who is being edged out of office because he keeps a mistress is to be replaced by a corrupt minister with no public spirit at all. Disraeli links the decline of party politics and rise of "political infidelity" and politics-as-theater with the reform bill; he suggests that the public, not competent to judge political careers, choose rather to judge the candidates' private characters, which can easily be smeared in public opinion through poster campaigns and like measures. In turn, the public is unable to weigh political issues. Egremont himself wins his campaign with the slogan "Vote for our young Queen and Egremont" against his opponent's "Vote for McDruggy and our young Queen" (71), rather than on the issues, which his opponent, who does attempt to take a position, quickly drops since his opinions are unpopular. Even the slogan comes not from Egremont but from Tadpole, the spin doctor. Laborers must have exemplary domestic lives to build "social happiness," but this is separate from the real business of state; laborers should remain in the domestic sphere, which ought to be separate from the public.[2]

2. Wahrman notes that the importance of the concept of "public opinion" in the late 1810s and early 1820s was "unprecedented" (190). He identifies public opinion with the public sphere in the work of Habermas and rebukes Habermas for his uncritical identification of public opinion with the middle classes and with reason. Wahrman is certainly correct in noting that public opinion was not necessarily narrowly bourgeois. But public opinion was often vilified, in the nineteenth century

This perhaps provides some explanation for Disraeli's ambiguous attitude toward women in politics. Women in Disraeli's novels are very active politically, which he seems to take as a matter of course. Egremont's successful campaign, and, indeed, the entire beginning of his political career, is managed by his mother, which Disraeli suggests is the natural course of events. Aristocratic women write leading articles on political topics for newspapers that guide public opinion (326) and control MPs' votes by offering them entry into "society" (327). Refusal of this kind of bait is represented as unusual. However, it is important to recall that Egremont becomes fitted for political life only after he takes office and has his eyes opened by contact with the oppressed Saxon, Gerard. Women's political interests are represented largely as both strategic and personally interested: they vie for power for themselves and their relatives, not to advance a political ideal. Egremont's mother gives him no political opinions, only an understanding of how the system can be manipulated for gain. And when the Tory ladies are balked by one who resists their social bait, Egremont uses the opportunity to tell them, "There is a lesson for you fine ladies, who think you can govern the world by what you call your social influences . . . [as] a reward for great exertions, or, if necessary, an inducement to infamous tergiversation" (327). The "social influence" of the ladies corrupts, by offering rewards that should be in the private sphere for public work, blending the two to the damage of the political process.

In short, Disraeli's politics, at least as he presents them to the public in the Young England novels of the mid-1840s, foreshadow the cultural liberalism of post-Chartist liberal writers such as Kingsley and Eliot in several themes, most notably, the importance of social welfare promoted through sanitary housing and the cultural elevation of the populace; individualism and liberty as opposed to direct political representation; the use of the raced body and narratives of national identity to ground a teleology of cultural progress; and, to a lesser extent, the need for a separation between public and private. Disraeli is somewhat unique in representing that division as far from present practice; however, this is probably in large part because his novels are not in the domestic tradition, which is where such a division is most emphatically celebrated. They tend to overlap with the tradition of the silver fork novels of the 1830s and 1840s and to portray aristocratic characters, as opposed to the middle-class characters (or those identified as such) of the domestic novel.

---

and now (including by Habermas himself), as the unreasoning emotional reaction of the mass—the opposite of the reasoned operations of the public sphere. In Disraeli we see public opinion feminized as quite the opposite of reasoned political debate.

Miss Marjoribanks: Managing Politics through the Social

The division between public and private was so emphatically and widely celebrated, in fact, that it lent itself to parody. Elizabeth Langland's superb reading of *Miss Marjoribanks* documents the way in which Oliphant dismantles the ideal of the domestic angel and of marriage, which the Carlingford heroines regard as stepping stones to a political career, after "seiz[ing] control of local society through dexterous manipulation of domestic discursive practices and a clever staging of class and femininity" (*Nobody's Angels* 156). Langland concludes that "it seems likely that middle-class feminism was forged, at least in part, in the smithy of women's social management, which gave women an inclination for professional work even as it taught them that they had the skills to pursue it" (ibid., 208). As she also points out, this particular form of feminism reinforced class boundaries between "sisters," rather than diminishing them: "middle-class feminism was built upon the assumption that another class existed to perform menial labor, and working-class women were constructed to bolster and facilitate the middle-class project" (ibid.).

Langland also observes, "Although the links between Society and politics are often occluded, the connection is tellingly exposed in the coincidence of the London 'Season' with the sitting of Parliament" (ibid., 31); it is the closer connection of society and politics that I would like to draw out here. I would like to build on Langland's evocative reading of *Miss Marjoribanks* to suggest that the humor of the Carlingford novels (which, it must be admitted, were by no means Oliphant's most popular—as Langland speculates, these probably cut too close to the bone to be heartily embraced by the public) is based on their satirical treatment of Victorian liberalism's positioning of middle-class women vis-à-vis the social. *Miss Marjoribanks* was published in 1866; the Second Reform Bill debates ran hot and heavy throughout the 1860s until the bill's passage in 1867, and by this time the porous relation of politics, domesticity, and the social could be the subject of wry commentary on women's power. Young Lucilla Marjoribanks aims, for most of the novel, to be "of help to her fellow creatures" through the medium of "Society"—that is, setting up her ideal of social life in Carlingford through the sponsorship of "Evenings," weekly dinner parties designed to draw middle-class Carlingford together and build community.[3]

3. Interestingly, when Trollope treats this same theme in *The Prime Minister*, he insists, like Egremont, that the days of social influences are over; moreover, he makes the failure of aristocratic and middle-class women to be sufficiently socially exclusive end disastrously for the men who govern Britain. Lady Glencora, ambitious of governing through dinner parties, is derided by the men who surround her, and she succeeds only in disgracing herself and her husband, the prime minister, by implying the promise of a political position to a man considered unsuited to hold it by class, ethnic

Oliphant pokes fun at the seriousness with which Lucilla takes her aims by defining her activities consistently throughout the entire novel in martial and political language: Lucilla does "battle," "retires with the full honours of war" (I.16), and takes "the reins of state" out of her father's hands. However, as we shall see, the novel also clearly indicates that there *is* crossover between the masculine world of politics—"Them" as Lucilla condescendingly refers to "the gentlemen"—and the feminine world of Lucilla's Evenings. Thus, the comic language becomes the language most simply factual in its description of the structure of power in Carlingford, and comedy based on satirizing the domestic novel insensibly blends into realism. The third volume of the novel makes the connection explicit, moving ahead to Lucilla's maturity. She enters her thirties as a liberal "statesman" (as the narrator often terms her), when she pilots one candidate safely into port as MP for Carlingford and sets out to marry and make another man a member for the county as well.

Teenaged Lucilla asks her school mistress to teach her "all about Political Economy and things, to help me manage everything" (I.16), and she returns to England feeling "more and more that she who held the reorganization of society in Carlingford in her hands was a woman with a mission. She was going abroad as the heir apparent went to America and the Holy Land, to complete her education, and fit herself, by an examination of the peculiarities of other nations, for an illustrious and glorious reign at home" (I.30). Her first suitor, slated to be future MP for Carlingford, congratulates her on her "social politics," which are "masterly," and cites her "statesmanlike views," telling her she "ought to be Prime Minister" (I.159). Lucilla's primary reason for considering his suit—which runs aground because of his attraction to a lower-middle-class woman whom Lucilla has brought to the dinner party because of her fine voice—is that "there was something in the very idea of being MP for Carlingford which moved the mind of Lucilla. It was a perfectly ideal position for a woman of her views, and seemed to offer the very field that was necessary for her ambition" (I.164). Typically, she regards the man who actually holds the position as an incidental annoyance necessary to her own rule. This foreshadows the moment in the third volume when she engineers his electoral defeat in favor of her own (new) candidate.

A liberal sovereign, alternatively described as an "enlightened despot" (I.61), Lucilla plans a limited expansion of the range of classes to be admitted to "society." As she says to the drawing master's daughter, whom she wants to sing at her evenings, "As for the ridiculous idea that nobody can be called on who does not live in Grange Lane, I assure you I mean to make an end of that" (I.59)—though it is worth pointing out that this inclusion

background (he is of Spanish parentage and may be Jewish), and economic position.

of a highly sexualized, lower-middle-class woman has nothing but disastrous results. Still, she has "all that regard for constituted rights which is so necessary to a revolutionary of the highest class" (I.139) and so mollifies the persons whom her new ways are challenging. Her religious and political opinions are strictly orthodox, without being extreme, for she has "no desire to shock anyone's prejudices" (ibid.). Langland points out that "The angel, or true English woman, works to make class a non-issue, relegating effects of nurture to the category of nature"—a mystifying rhetoric in which the middle-class woman becomes the naturally maternalistic superior of lower-class women (*Nobody's Angels* 76). Yet at the same time, the novel is entirely attentive to class difference, which, as Langland points out, was a key issue for middle-class women. They were charged with the task of mastering the "signifying practices" of upper- and upper-middle-class life, performing them and policing the boundaries to keep out "undesirables"—that is, those who had not mastered those practices (ibid., 25–26).

The novel does indeed rigidly police class boundaries, and, as Langland argues, it depicts a heroine deploying a rhetoric of social distinction to leverage power. We should also note here, however, that this social power is to be leveraged for the good of all in a way that is distinctly and directly political in structure and, eventually, in nature. Additionally, the ultimate goal of her politics is to eradicate the significance of class distinctions—as she tells the lower-middle-class woman whom she invites to her parties, not all at once, but eventually, she will break class barriers down. Class resentment, however, works against this liberal project, and, as Lucilla's first suitor points out, the young woman does not have the social skills to benefit from this relaxation of social boundaries. She is, he tells Lucilla, "charming raw material; but if I were you, I would put her through an elementary course. If you make a pretty-behaved young woman out of that, you will beat Adam Smith" (I.159). Lucilla retorts that she did not read Smith, who was "rather old-fashioned," but he is right—though that does not stop him from becoming romantically entangled with this inadequately socialized creature. Finally, Lucilla recognizes that the middle classes do not take instruction very well, intent on "freezing each other" by upholding their petty differences in privilege; it is the poor who will provide her with a relatively malleable "raw material" whose abilities to interact socially can be radically improved.

The comedy of the novel emerges from the transgression of the boundaries between the social and the political, the private and the public; the nervousness of that humor is based on the novel's demonstration of the transparent fictitiousness of that distinction. As opposed to comedies based on gender transgression—which the novel gestures toward, for example, in portraying

Lucilla as a large and therefore somewhat masculinized woman—the real humor comes from the characters' strict adherence to gender roles and the implication that a reversal of "normal" power relations is implicit within those roles themselves. Lucilla is a perfect lady, unconcerned about politics, committed to being "a comfort to Papa" and helping her "fellow creatures" with her domestic and social skills—and in so doing, she aspires to rule England and, not incidentally, arranges the lives of the "inferior creatures" who dutifully, if clumsily, fulfill their appointed masculine parts.

Lucilla's suitors represent all ranks of good society and its governance, but all fail not only to win her but even to woo her (they are all somehow stopped in the very act of proposing). The end of the parliamentary hopeful we have already seen. He has sexual habits that will not bear scrutiny and is satisfyingly physically degenerate when he returns from the continent ten years after his suit of Lucilla fails; he has grown fat and looks old (as Lucilla puts it, he has "gone off"). One by one the other suitors go to women who are lower in status than Lucilla. From the failed future MP, the narrative turns to a "Broad Church" potential bishop. But the Kingsleyan Muscular Christian archdeacon is too broad for Lucilla; "he just as often agreed with the gentlemen in their loose ways of thinking, as with the more correct opinions by which the wives and mothers who had charge of Their morality strove hard to keep them in the right way" (I.247). He marries a middle-class widow whom Lucilla had taken up as an object of charity, a woman whom he loves intensely but does not respect at all. Next, a general does not get very far, as he is attracted to the (quite respectable but still unacceptably lower-middle-class) sister of the woman who derailed the first suitor. A doctor who courts her ends up with a "little Australian" he is "crazy about." In three of these cases, Lucilla actually engineers the marriages of the men whose taste is so "unfortunate." Only the last, the candidate whom she steers into office as member for Carlingford, and whom she is about to accept, is really ready to marry her, yet she chooses her cousin instead, prompting the narrator to remark that it is a comfort that Lucilla will not have to change her name.

In fact, it is quite clear throughout that Lucilla is not much interested in any of these men but rather in the exercise of power that they may provide—they each represent a different branch of the key professions. At the moment she is giving up the Broad Church archdeacon to his former love interest, she is, in fact, delighted, for "it did her heart good to take the management of incapable people, and arrange all their affairs for them, and solve all their difficulties. Such an office was more in her way than all the Archdeacons in the world" (II.79).[4] Miss Marjoribanks wishes to rule people "all for [their]

4. In this sense, Lucilla is a bit like Austen's Emma in reverse. As in *Emma,* the comedy comes

own good" (II.172); the love and marriage plot memorialized by Nancy Armstrong is overturned with a vengeance, as Miss Marjoribanks marries not even for the money that represents indirect political power for women but for that power itself.

Male characters in the novel often fail to see the novel's women as individuals, usually with the result that women are easily able to manipulate them. Lucilla's first homecoming "roused [the Doctor] for the first time to consider his little girl as a creature possessed of individual character" (I.13), and he views her with such dismay that he sends her back to school for three more years and to the Continent for another. Most men, however, move through their lives without recognizing women's rather dangerous individuality and remain largely oblivious to the social structures that organize their lives, for "in delicate matters of social politics, one never expects to be understood by *them*"—that is, men (I.179, emphasis in original).

On the other hand, the novel suggests that "They" are not so individual as they think they are. Lucilla challenges the gentlemen who provide "the background" of her Evenings, "Never mind what he is like; you gentlemen can never describe anybody—you always keep to *generals*" (I.271, emphasis in original). She turns the tables on the usual claim that women cannot think in abstract terms by suggesting that the men think so generally as to be, unknowingly, massified. The Broad Churchman, whose views of women are much like Kingsley's, is described as "one of those men who are very strong for the masculine side of Christianity" (I.253), who demands a great deal of attention and deference from women that he is not willing to pay in turn. Any woman he approves of is defined as "'a good, pure, gentle woman.' . . . He spoke in a tone which settled the question . . . and no doubt what he said was perfectly true, though it was not a very distinct characterization" (II.58); good women are not individuals for him. The woman he "loved better than anything else in the world" has no opinion that had "the weight of a straw upon him" (II.258). Oliphant chooses him to be the character most humiliated—for his own good, of course—by Lucilla's abilities. Constrained not to denounce an enemy at her party, he is "in a state of repression and restraint, which it was painful, and at the same time pleasing, to see. . . . Such are the beneficial restraints of society, that he dared not follow his natural impulses . . . for fear of Miss Marjoribanks, which was about the highest testimony to the value of social influence that can be given" (II.246–47). By the end of his

from the complacency of the managing woman; however, unlike Austen's heroine, who must learn the inappropriateness of her self-estimation through bitter humiliation, Lucilla's wisdom and ability is confirmed, not only by her final success in managing her own affairs but also by the beneficial arrangement of everyone else's.

narrative, Lucilla "knew in her heart that the Archdeacon was afraid of her" (II.268).

It is hardly surprising, then, when in the third volume Lucilla turns directly to politics. When the old MP for Carlingford dies, she selects a new one. Here again, she shows a fine liberal sense of the importance of public opinion. Declining to hear his detailed political statement, she instructs him not to worry about political questions, since she sees no difference between Whigs or Tories: "Don't go making speeches about opinions. If you begin with that, there's no end to it. . . . I know what you gentlemen are" (III.16). The important thing, she assures him, is that he is "the right man" for Carlingford, and this tribute to liberal individualism works in the novel to convince voters who are diametrically opposed to him politically; they are persuaded to judge him as a citizen, a neighbor and consumer, rather than evaluating his politics. After all, Lucilla points out, "when it comes to doing anything, the Whigs and Tories are just the same. Mr. Ashburton, it is the Man that is wanted" (III.19). (Here she echoes the wisdom of Disraeli's Tadpole.) Her candidate laughs when Lucilla assures him that the most important thing is to pick the color of his ribbons, but as usual, she is right. Public opinion is indeed feminized. Lucilla galvanizes the town's women, who "in no cases had votes; but Miss Marjoribanks, with instinctive correctness of judgment, decided that there were more things to be thought of than the electors" (III.24).

What wins the election, it is suggested, is a combination of popular feeling against the sexual morals of the opposition and the dissenting shopkeepers, "who . . . decided for the man who 'dealt' in George Street"—that is, consumed locally (III.222). In short, the women who control social politics and the domestic economics of the candidates' own households and their impact on the private economic lives of the voters control the outcome of politics in Carlingford. As for issues, the most exciting question in politics at the time was reform, but this was the 1860s, not the 1830s, so even the grocer, "Mr. Tozer [who] had once been in a dreadful state of mind about . . . It [Reform] was quite tranquil on the subject now, and so was the community in general" (III.73); Tozer votes for Lucilla's more conservative candidate on the basis of the candidate's standing in the community and continuing trade at his store. Oliphant offers a tableau during a comic scene in which the opposing candidates, both sometime suitors of Lucilla, meet in her drawing room and she smoothes over the awkwardness: "she stood between them a picture of angelic sweetness and goodness, giving a certain measure of her sympathy to both—Woman the Reconciler, by the side of those other characters of Inspirer and Consoler, of which the world has heard. The two inferior creatures scowled . . . at each other, but Miss Marjoribanks smiled upon them both" (III.85). Here

Lucilla not only rules the community but *is* the community being courted by opposing candidates, who herself, as "society," recognizes that community building is more important in the 1860s than politics. Thus, feminized "society" trumps Parliament as a locus of power, even though Lucilla "had come to an age at which she might have gone into parliament herself, had there been no disqualification of sex, and when it was almost a necessity for her to make some use of her social influence" (III.85). In a Romney Leigh–like moment, looking for projects, she even briefly considers marrying a poor man in order to make him over and provide a moral example to society at large.

When Lucilla's father dies and she is left relatively poor herself, the local clergyman comes to indicate that parish work is the "proper sphere" for Lucilla, since she is unmarried (III.178). This endeavor has little immediate appeal. Still, once Lucilla becomes engaged, she begins to pair the notion of social work with political power as she considers that she may make her fiancé an MP for the county after they move to a country house associated with her ancestral name. Thus, she unites the urban professional class (as a doctor's daughter) and the old feudal notion of the rural lady of the manor so dear to readers of Carlyle and Ruskin. Lucilla's organization of "society," which dominates the first two volumes of the novel, is early on connected to the larger domain of the social, which foreshadows her ultimate commitment to social work. As she is on her way to prepare for the first dinner party she will give in Carlingford, she is accosted by a female beggar with many children. She does not give money, as that is contrary to her education in political economy, but she offers to find the woman work (which the narrator assures us will rid her of any further importunities by the impoverished family), because "Lucilla, to do her justice, felt it equally natural that beneficence should issue from her in this manner as in that other mode of feeding the hungry which she had solemnly engaged herself to fulfil at seven o'clock"—that is, giving a dinner party (93). She also aids the "decayed gentlewoman" who eventually marries the Broad Churchman, providing her with a place to live and a school.

So the reader is prepared when the mature Lucilla considers that social work with the poor will be more satisfying than her quite similar work with "society." Her work as a society hostess, it is suggested, is simply training for this larger and nobler project. Besides, despite vows of "protection and guidance from the strong to the weak . . . uttered in . . . [her] liberal heart," society is not grateful, nor does it learn to replicate for itself the skills she has modeled:

> "After working at it for ten years! . . . they will go back to their old ridiculous parties, as if they had never seen anything better; and they will all break up

> into little cliques, and make their awful morning calls and freeze one another to death . . . after one has slaved like a—woman in a mill" said the disappointed reformer . . . "But the poor . . . could not help being better for what one did for them. They might continue to be as stupid as ever, and ungrateful . . . but if they were warm and comfortable, instead of cold and hungry, it would always make a difference." (III.270–71)

Sanitary reform, which she had rejected when suggested by the two clergy who advocate it in the novel, suddenly becomes attractive: "There are people who are very tragical about village nuisances, and there are other people who assail them with loathing . . . but Lucilla [had] . . . the liveliest satisfaction to think of all the disorder and disarray. . . . Her fingers itched to be at it" (III.276). Characteristic of the period, sanitary reform is conceived both as the legislative elimination of nuisances and as housing reform, with a good deal of tutelage thrown in: "Lucilla's eyes went over the moral wilderness with the practical glance of a statesman, and, at the same time, the sanguine enthusiasm of a philanthropist" (III.291). With a "vision of a parish saved, a village reformed, a county reorganised, and a triumphant election . . . which should put the government of the country itself, to a certain extent, into competent hands," she sees a "larger sphere opening out" wherein she can serve "her generation in a twofold way, among the poor and among the rich" (III.293) to whom she shall carry "light and progress" (III.296).

Lucilla sees the reformation and organization of the poor as a clear extension of her activities as a society hostess and, in turn, in a series of local to general displacements much like Octavia Hill's rhetoric of social duty, this reorganization as the first step in governing the country through better organization and a maternal care for people's "own good." Significantly, this is all embodied in the notion of sanitary reform, which encapsulates all these hopes. As we saw earlier in the novel, there is no suggestion that economic hardship causes poverty—the beggar who asks for money is offered work, and the people of the village are offered education and housing reform. Interestingly, however, we see some rebellion against this ideal. The upper-class members of society rebel against Lucilla's dominion—despite Lucilla's beneficent influence, when her father dies and she withdraws from society, their relief is described as revolutionary, a "republican" pleasure in "liberty" (III.152)—and the poor are expected to be "ungrateful" as well. And of course, Oliphant satirizes her heroine, reminding us often of how unbearable her presumptuousness can be. But Oliphant is ambivalent on this score: Lucilla is represented as genuinely kind, self-sacrificing, concerned about others, and, most important, successful in promoting their happiness and welfare, even against their will. Where Lucilla fails, it is because of forces working against enlightenment reason: "even the aid of Miss Marjoribanks was as nothing against dead selfishness and folly, the two most invincible forces in the world" (II.291).

The novel responds to the domestic tradition so ably described by Armstrong, satirizing, though gently, the sense of middle-class women's self-importance that Dickens savages in characters such as Mrs. Pardiggle and Mrs. Jellyby, the female philanthropists of *Bleak House.* Yet, finally, Oliphant is even harder on male self-importance about public life, which is shown to be peripheral to real-life issues and entirely dependent on the feminized and female-dominated domestic and social realm, wherein liberal government actually takes place and both political decisions and effective improvements are actually made. The iron hand in Miss Marjoribanks's size large velvet glove, it is intimated, will rule England, eventually, with the same "enlightened despotism," on the same liberal principles, economic, moral, and social, that she learned at her finishing school, and used in conducting "society" in Grange Lane—and much the better for everyone, into the bargain, than the foolishness of Whigs and Tories who blather endlessly about reform, which comes to nothing.

As is typical in liberal rhetoric as diverse as Kingsley's, Eliot's, Arnold's, and Mill's—and even Disraeli's (whose eccentric Young Englandism surely rests on a foundation of liberal rhetoric in respect to values, despite its political nostalgia for a grand Toryism and monarchic rule), access to the franchise is seen as signifying little; what really matters is "light," "progress," and educational and sanitary reform that will create the potential for the development of the enlightened subjects of a liberal society. Significantly, after Lucilla receives, with little enthusiasm, the clergyman's suggestion that she do parish work, it is a lower-middle-class woman who points the way. Rose, a woman artist who early in the novel advocates art schools as a kind of Ruskinian cultural program of enlightenment for the poor, has lost faith in art by the end of the novel; still, she advises Lucilla to adopt a typically feminine approach to social work—she should "mother" the poor and teach them "how to live and how to manage" (III.177). When Lucilla thinks about it in these terms, as an extension of domestic management and the fostering of proper subjects of society, the sanitary work she despises earlier in the novel and associates with the Broad Churchman suddenly becomes much more appealing.

Early on in the novel, Lucilla makes the domestic sphere the basis of her reign. As in Godwin's discussion of the home decorating of the poor, aesthetics are a key element of social control: Lucilla manages on her first night home from school to redecorate the drawing room with her personal items, a "fundamental duty of woman" (I.47) that makes the room "an individual spot of ground revealing something of the character of its mistress"; within the first two weeks she has redecorated and reupholstered with fabric to set off her looks, seeing the room as a kind of dress, and confusing the upholsterer by holding up drapery to her face to see how well it harmonizes with her skin. Oliphant is, of course, satirizing the language of the conduct manuals Lucilla has consulted in planning her takeover, but Lucilla is also correct. The drawing room is an extension of the woman's dress, in fact, of her classed body (as one sees clearly in Gaskell's *North and South,* for example).

As in *Bleak House,* wherein the domestic goddess Esther's every detail of household management is replicated by grateful men, who take it from a London suburb to a Yorkshire village, Lucilla's metastasizing domestic influence is replicated in the country house near Carlingford when her fiancé goes to the upholsterer and demands for the Marchbank estate the exact same green fabric with which Lucilla dressed her first drawing room. Whereas Dickens's domestic and social ideal represents a site of sanctuary from the world of politics and bureaucracy, however, Oliphant's ambivalent satire positions Lucilla's drawing room (or "throne," as the narrator terms it) as the very epicenter of political power. It is, after all, Lucilla's drawing-room colors, green and lavender, that are worn by the party of the winning MP for Carlingford.

Lucilla's mode of organizing knowledge is the epitome of governmentality. She combines the theoretical knowledge learnt in conduct books and at school, where she prepares herself in political economy and moral philosophy, with the experiential knowledge learned on her grand tour, and puts this knowledge to work using her good instincts for the talents of the persons surrounding her, whom she regards as tools. She values theoretic knowledge yet scorns slavish devotion to the mere generalities "they" are capable of, in favor of intimate knowledge of the individuals she must work with. Her ten-year apprenticeship in local management prepares her for the "larger sphere" of the county—and the country. Oliphant folds the political novel into the domestic novel seamlessly—and can do so, she suggests, because the difference between the two domains is largely imaginary anyway.

8

THE SOCIAL NOVEL'S LEAKY BODIES

> There is not a drop of Tom's polluted blood but propagates infection and contagion somewhere. There is not an Atom of Tom's slime . . . but shall work its retribution, through every order of society.
>
> —Charles Dickens, *Bleak House*

> They carried a door, taken off its hinges, upon their shoulders, upon which lay some dead human creature; . . . all might see the poor drowned wretch—his glassy eyes, one half open, staring right upwards to the sky.
>
> —Elizabeth Gaskell, *North and South*

Bodily Fluids

Having sketched out a broad context for the political novel and its relations to the social in the period, I would like to examine the representation of the desiring body in the mid-Victorian liberal novel. Just as mid-century liberals promoted a form of social citizenship that was only potentially related to political representation, so many of these novels concerned themselves primarily with the social. These novels avoided direct representations of politics but were preoccupied with social questions such as poverty, disease, and crime, and these questions were thematized through the portrayal of the body. Herbert Sussman has traced in detail Carlyle's use of images of liquidity and pulpiness to describe the unformed masculine self, which only careful self-cultivation and control would enclose in a relatively firm and clearly defined structure. He relates these images specifically to Carlyle's understanding of masculinity. I would like to suggest that this imagery was actually fairly pervasive in mid-Victorian culture (though Carlyle certainly gave it his own inimitable twist). Rather than the raw and the cooked, one might think of Victorian social oppositions as often being defined as the opposition between liquid and solid, wet and dry. Cholera, of course, literalized this undisciplined evacuation of fluids and linked it to the uncontained human fluids associated with improper drainage, mapping the individual onto the built environment. But this was simply one powerful model of a more widely held understanding of the dangers that uncontrolled physicality held for the social body. Individuality, not exclusively masculine but certainly masculinized, was based on a model of the body that contained and separated itself from the bodies of others, but the sick, undisciplined body threatened to sink the individual into the unreasoning mass of continuous, imbruted embodiment.

The pulpiness within the dangerous body was always threatening to burst the bounds of the skin, which defined and disciplined individual embodiment. Disease, lack of self-control, femininity, and madness were all aligned with liquidity, liquefaction, and perhaps putrefaction as well—those who lacked self-control and possessive individualism were liable to melt back into a primal flow of dangerous ooze. Just as, as Armstrong argues, the threat of political combination was coded as sexual scandal in the narratives of the late 1840s and early 1850s, disruption in the social body was coded as a lack of discipline rendered literally as a lack of self-containment. In women this was indeed often figured as inappropriate sexual openness; in men it was often aligned with tropes of addiction and plot lines involving mass violence. But in either case, fluidity often grounded descriptions of the body disintegrating as a threat to the larger social body.

North and South: Redirecting Desire

Gaskell's *North and South* provides a convenient example of this dichotomy in an 1850s liberal novel. Gaskell carefully eschews direct political commentary, handling even political economy with disclaimers in order to focus on social effects of economic hardship. This classic tale of class conflict has long been used to illustrate Raymond Williams's thesis; like *Mary Barton* before it, this novel creates a narrative of class struggle that then calls upon a middle-class love story as a solution that many critics say elides the first narrative entirely. Others, following Armstrong, have pointed out that the novel actually uses the courtship plot as a way to reshape subjectivity in the novel, building a bond of sympathy between the classes based on a shared vision of bourgeois personhood. I would like to expand on this reading to discuss the role of depictions of the body in identifying a correctly embodied (masculine, middle-class) subjectivity.

Images of liquidity combine with those of inappropriate domesticity and privacy. The culmination of class tension that is about to erupt into a riot (as is usual in the factory novels of the late 1840s and early 1850s) is figured as a flood: Margaret feels the "thunderous atmosphere, morally as well as physically" and sees the massing of the inhabitants in the streets as an illicit use of public space: "From every narrow lane . . . came up a low distant roar. . . . The inhabitants of each poor squalid dwelling were gathered around the doors and windows, if indeed they were not standing in the middle of the narrow ways." She hears the "first far-off roll of the tempest;—saw the first slow surging wave of the dark crowd come, with its threatening crest, tumble over, and retreat" (170). This flood is stopped short of actual riot when Margaret, shielding Thornton, is struck by a stone and bleeds: the crowd is "watching, open-eyed and open-mouthed, the thread of dark red blood which wakened them up from their trance of passion . . . the tears welled out of the long entanglement of eyelashes, and dropped down, and heavier, slower splash than even tears, came the drip of blood from her wound. Even the most desperate—Boucher himself—drew back, faltered away" (178).

Margaret's public display of her body, of course, is figured as a small sexual scandal, being read by Thornton's family as a declaration of love for him. But what halts the crowd is not the spectacle of sexual desire that the Thorntons see—the workers believe her to be Thornton's sister—but the spectacle of her vulnerability, marked by the escape of fluid from her body, which is supposed to be superbly closed and invulnerable, shielded by both her gender and her class. One kind of flood is, temporarily, at least, held off by a counterflow of small size but immense significance. If the middle-class woman's body disintegrates, then, truly, the social body collapses.[1]

It is important to note, however, that Gaskell builds sympathy for this frightening and dangerous deluge of working-class rage by making the cause of it the destruction of their domestic sphere by economic forces. Although the narrator bows to Thornton's declaration that the misery of the workers is caused by lack of self-restraint, the narrative dwells on the misery of starving children and hungry wives (this emphasis was even more pronounced in her earlier novel *Mary Barton,* wherein we see the house slowly stripped of dishes, furniture, and finally even fire for the hearth as the poverty of the family progresses). Thus, the rage of the factory workers is made intelligible, as is their loss of self-control—it is motivated by the loss of secure boundaries in the very base of that control, the family and home itself. If they gather not only in

1. Ironically, Margaret is at the Thorntons' home seeking a waterbed, contained fluid for the relief of the dying body of her mother.

their "squalid dwellings" but in the "narrow ways," Gaskell suggests, perhaps it is not because they are not capable of recognizing the difference between home and street but because any meaningful distinction between them has been erased.

Boucher is the stereotype of the undisciplined worker—a man with many children whose nerve fails as soon as they begin to cry for food. His gradual loss of self-control is marked first by his own tears, then by unleashing the "storm" of the riot, and finally by bloodletting (he has led the riot in which Margaret is injured; later he will bloody the face of the union leader, Higgins, who curses him for the loss of self-control that alienates the public and destroys the strike). Boucher's lack of self-containment is marked by his Irishness, his large, dirty, undisciplined family, and his inability to provide for them; he is a pauper in the making. Finally, the body whose seams have leaked so portentously gives way entirely; Boucher's disintegration is emblematized, literally and shockingly, by the actual liquefaction of his drowned and waterlogged body. When Margaret accuses Higgins and the union of, through exerting pressure to strike on Boucher, having "made him what he is!" the line immediately following underscores the question of identity:

> made him what he is! What was he? . . . They carried a door, taken off its hinges, upon their shoulders, upon which lay some dead human creature; and from each side of the door there were constant droppings. . . . All might see the poor drowned wretch—his glassy eyes, one half open, staring right upwards to the sky. . . . His face was swollen and discoloured; besides, his skin was stained by the water in the brook, which had been used for dyeing purposes. . . . The hair grew long and thin behind, and every separate lock was a conduit for water. (288)

Boucher's body, bereft of privacy, becomes an object for the public gaze as Margaret's was. The water, contaminated by industrial by-products, is a fit image of the economic pressures and social irresponsibility that combine with Boucher's lack of self-control to dissolve his fragile selfhood.

As Heather Milton argues, Boucher is a foil for Higgins. Milton notes that Margaret, as middle-class woman, not only humanizes Thornton and renders him more sympathetic but also fosters the development of middle-class masculinity in Higgins. Higgins already has elements of middle-class subjectivity for Margaret to build on; he compares his relation to the union to that of a soldier's to the nation. Defending the strike, he argues that he "'look[s] forward to the chance of dying at my post sooner than yield. That's what folk call fine and honorable in a soldier, and why not in a poor-weaver chap?'" Margaret argues that a soldier dies "in the cause of the Nation—in the cause of others," whereupon he answers that he, too, sacrifices in the cause of others and of justice—and of others he knows, rather than "somebody he never clapt eyes on" (134). His error, for Margaret, is that he considers loyalty to his order to be comparable to loyalty to the nation. Still, the notion of self-sacrifice in the service of a larger aim is one, for Margaret, of which something may be made. The rhetoric is quite close to that of the reform bill debates several years later; workers have proven the capacity of loyalty to some overarching aim by proving capable of combination, and now that nascent capacity for public identity must be turned toward citizenship rather than class.

As Octavia Hill emphasizes, public spirit arises first out of a commitment to local community—here, as Higgins says, to John Boucher's cause. Mr. Hale, representing the liberal's reluctant admiration for such disciplined self-sacrifice, sighs, "Your Union would be beautiful, glorious,—it would be Christianity itself—if it were but for an end which affected the good of all, instead of that of merely one class as opposed to another" (229). If combination is, as Armstrong posits, a terrifying scandal, it is also the very basis of liberal citizenship. The question is how to turn it from the too "massive" class-based combination to a suitably "individualized" understanding of citizenship. Higgins takes that first step when he offers to undercut ditchdiggers' wages in order to gain work to support the children he has adopted. Though the Hales point out to him that he would be a "knobstick" himself if he did that, he actually drops the plan simply because it is unworkable. In putting family first, before his class affiliation and his union, he takes the first step toward a bourgeois notion of possessive individualism.

Patrick Brantlinger notes the Unitarian Gaskell's debt to Christian Socialism, its optimism and presentation of economic suffering as a necessary spiritual test on the way to brighter futures (*Spirit* 141–42). Still, he notes, she does not fall into the Manichean and unworkable oppositions or the utopian predictions of Kingsley and his ilk. Higgins is not made simply to renounce his ethical commitment to the union but to reorganize the priority of his commitments. The disorder introduced into the weakest tissue of the social body by the strike provides a terrible object lesson. Although the small breach of Margaret's body stops the worst of the mass violence, Boucher's death symbolizes the dangers of class consciousness to the masses who do not have the self-control Higgins has. Although he and others like him did not authorize Boucher's violence, they bear the responsibility for mobilizing a segment of society not sufficiently self-contained to manage their own bodies (though

Boucher manages sufficient discipline to drown himself, very deliberately, in very little water). Bloated, blackened, made racially other, he is still recognizable "through all these disfigurements" (288) as a member of Higgins's community whose vulnerability is made as horrifyingly clear as Margaret's is by her "splashing" blood.

Higgins's taking up of "John Boucher's cause" has done Boucher no favors, having "made of him what he is"; misplaced, overly local, public spiritedness kills. The shock of this sight and his feeling of responsibility for Boucher's fate drive Higgins to take responsibility for Boucher's children, forcing him to set aside union activity in order to get work. Margaret had already persuaded Higgins to stop drinking—another sign of both his lower-class status and his lack of physical self-control. This new manifestation of his character leads Margaret to remark that there are "'grand makings of a man . . . in him. . . . There's granite in all these northern people,'" to which her father replies that there was "none in poor Boucher" or his wife. Margaret dismissively responds that "they had Irish blood" (301–2), racializing the boundary line between the potential citizen and the pauper. Stone and metal are the substances persistently opposed to the dangerous liquidity of the masses in Gaskell's novel; one might think of John Ruskin's and Walter Pater's persistent use of mineral imagery for masculinity and selfhood.

Higgins's first response to the shock of Boucher's death shows his development as a middle-class subject when compared to his earlier reactions to disappointments. His response to the failures of the workers' plans is to seek companionship at the pub. When his daughter dies, earlier in the story, he weeps and then attempts to go to the pub, but Margaret blocks the door, keeping him within his own house, policing the boundary between private grief and public display. When he does leave with her, it is to go drink tea with her father, and he avoids the gaze and conversation of his sympathetic neighbors. His reaction to Boucher's death is to bolt his door and attempt to be alone. Mr. Hale—a figure who represents the self-containment problems of the upper-class male—tries to insist on offering comfort, but Margaret, always the bearer of appropriate subjectivity in the novel, recognizes and approves this more private response to sorrow: "'I don't wonder at it. . . . I myself long to be alone'" (293). Higgins withdraws from the too-continuous local community to emphasize his individuality and solitude; instead of taking comfort in others of his class and in intoxicants, he will draw on the inner resources of a nascent middle-class interiority that he has earlier demonstrated in giving up the comforts of the pub for the comforts of reasoned debate with Mr. Hale.

Margaret sets great store in the effect of such reasoned discourse and conversation and attempts to promote it between masters and men. Such communication, she believes, will lead the workers from "childhood" into a potential adult citizenship. She accuses Thornton, a strong believer in possessive individualism who refuses to bother with any such tutelary communication, of wanting his workers to be like "tall, large children" (119), when she herself believes that these men are indeed children, but children in the awkward stage of transitioning to manhood. He responds, "'Well, in the Platonic year, it may fall out that we are all—men, women and children—fit for a republic: but give me a constitutional monarchy in our present state of morals and intelligence. . . . I agree with Miss Hale so far as to consider our people in the condition of children. . . . I maintain that despotism is the best kind of government for them'" (120). This despotism, however, is only for working hours; he disavows any responsibility for his workers once they are on their own time.

Margaret and Mr. Hale do not disagree with his assessment of the workers' present state but take the more progressive liberal position that the workers' moral "minority" implies a responsibility for moral guidance extending beyond the workday. Mr. Hale suggests that "a wise parent humours the desire for independent action, so as to become the friend and adviser when his absolute rule shall cease" (121). Taking the maternalistic position of the social, Margaret urges a gentle tutelage based on reasoned communication and "friendship" with the workers in their homes. Adult reason and self-control must be fostered by a maternal care such as Thornton has enjoyed himself. As Margaret says early on, she dislikes his "quietly professing to despise people for careless, wasteful improvidence, without ever seeming to think it his duty to try to make them different,—to give them anything of the training which his mother gave him, and to which he evidently owes his position" (87). Thornton here subscribes to a rather Aristotelian model of the citizen: power belongs by right to those who have mastered themselves and others—for the rest, submission. However, as one might expect of a man whose claim to public respect rests on his labor, he himself later repudiates the Greek model: "we are of a different race from the Greeks, to whom beauty was everything. . . . I belong to Teutonic blood. . . . We do not look upon life as a time for enjoyment, but as a time for action and exertion. Our glory and our beauty arise out of our inward strength, which makes us victorious over material resistance. . . . We stand up for self-government, and oppose centralization" (326).

Here is Carlylean liberalism that extends to all the possibility of becoming fit for citizenship but bases this fitness on mastery of "material resistance" that is also a continuing mastery of the body. Carlyle's model, however, grants to all men this capacity: in recognizing and following a leader who has such mastery, one comes to master oneself, and each individual rules his own private life, in turn becoming capable of participating in public "self-government." Carlyle's view also focuses on the continual struggle against a recalcitrant materiality (and embodiment) rather than on the liberation from materiality emphasized by Greek models of self-mastery. Both Thornton and the Hales adopt a strong liberal position, but Thornton's is one primarily of a negative liberty, whereas the Hales espouse a more intrusive state whose pedigree extends from Smith through Bentham and Mill. Thornton is forced, however, to reevaluate his self-contradictory commitment to a Herbert Spencerian possessive individualism when he faces the problem of the Other. "Despotism" is proper for the truly Other, but despotism implies responsibility. He abdicates responsibility on the basis of the workers' ability to elevate themselves to his own status, if they so choose—in which case, despotism is inappropriate and the problem of tutelary preparation for citizenship becomes paramount.

When Thornton finally succumbs to Margaret's influence and institutes reforms, he begins by providing an economical lunch service, replicating a domestic atmosphere in the workplace. Having been invited by the men to the table, he forms friendships with them, bonding in their common humanity in the act of fulfilling a bodily need. (It is important to point out that this service is not pauperizing; it is paid for entirely by the men's subscriptions, and so is consonant with liberal economics as well.) It is at these functions that he begins to build a communicative relationship with the men, encouraging them to make suggestions and giving them information about the workings of the business. Empowered by this Habermasian ideal, the workers respond with loyalty to the company, secretly working overtime to help Thornton.

Ironically, even this cannot undo the damage of the strike, for which Thornton pays by losing his business. However, he learns what Octavia Hill will believe to be central to her project thirty years later: "no mere institutions, however wise, . . . can attach class to class as they should be attached, unless the working out of such institutions bring the individuals of the different classes into actual personal contact. Such intercourse is the very breath of life" (421). Margaret approves of this speech so much that she offers him her inheritance to fund his next venture, which, of course, precipitates the final stamp of approval—she marries this fully socialized man, offering both her skills as a bourgeois homemaker (which have been favorably compared in several scenes to his nouveau riche mother's paint-by-numbers approach to creating a luxurious, but cold and uncomfortable, home) and their corollary, her talents as a social missionary.

Emerging from the Soggy Mass: *Bleak House,* Desire, and Domestic Fiction

As Dror Wahrman notes, political literature of the early nineteenth century insisted on the bourgeoisie's undomestic, too economic nature, but the novel and conduct books for women promoted the view of the domestic bourgeoisie, and it is certainly this view that prevailed in the bourgeois social imaginary by the mid-1830s. (By the late 1830s, the vision of the middle class promoted in fiction dominated political discourse as well.) By the 1860s, however, this now-hegemonic vision of bourgeois social subjectivity and the place of the woman within it had garnered significant critiques: one, a nascent feminist critique of the division between public and private (as we have seen with Mrs. Oliphant's *Miss Marjoribanks*); two, a protest against the power of the bourgeois woman as social missionary to cross the boundaries between the domestic and social-as-public sphere (as can be seen in Dickens's Mrs. Pardiggle and Mrs. Jellyby, the female philanthropists satirized in *Bleak House*); and three, sensation plots (such as *Lady Audley's Secret* or the Lady Dedlock plot in *Bleak House,* which suggest that the Lady Bountiful at the heart of this vision of the social is, as a woman, potentially a site of disorder and class transgression). The first two stressed the fictitiousness of the public-private divide, though they came to different conclusions about its desirability, but the third strikes at the heart of the icon of domesticity itself. The critical trend would continue in the 1870s, with the move toward the French-style realism of George Gissing and with the explosion of boy's and men's adventure novels and novels of empire, with their complex negotiation of the social as either hostile to men's imperial aims or, conversely, more appropriately administered by men than women. We cannot examine all of these possibilities here, but I would like to pursue a few of them.

Gaskell's novel, though published in 1855, reaches back to its 1848 companion novel, *Mary Barton.* In that sense, the novel has more to do with the direct political commentary of Disraeli than with the later social commentary of, say, Oliphant. Dickens's 1850s and 1860s novels are perhaps more in line with her time frame, in which the urgency of even indirect political commentary is muted and in which social commentary and the exploration of individual psychology becomes more central. In Dickens social problems are radically divorced from political questions; political solutions to social problems are not even an issue in his novels, whereas they still are by implication in Gaskell. Citizenship in Dickens is purely social citizenship, or participation in society as an appropriately desiring subject. However, as do Gaskell's, his novels appeal to the iconography of leakage versus containment in the service of a notion of liberal individualism, and to the healthy body as the basis for responsible social participation. He uses themes of sexual openness to indicate lack of self-containment in women and stories of addiction and its psychological double, obsession, to symbolize this same lack in men (and sometimes women as well). Both of these representations address desire out of control. The character who succumbs to these dangers fully risks losing individual identity and falling back into the status of mass, being part of an undifferentiated humanity that finally loses even its status as human. Conversely, those who succeed do so precisely by establishing an individual identity that is not *too* individual—not eccentric, but fully socialized—the good citizen, the good housewife. These are the characters who appropriately manage desire and whose bodies balance liquidity and containment.

John Kucich, in his perceptive *Excess and Restraint: The Novels of Charles Dickens,* has traced this dichotomy in several of Dickens's novels, including *Bleak House.* He reads the relationship as one between the formlessness of death and the conservative impulse toward life. Following Georges Bataille, he understands the novels as staging death—through loss, deaths, monetary excess, and the like—in order ultimately to recuperate order and restraint. Thus, the loss of Lady Dedlock becomes the way for Esther to integrate herself through "acceptable" versions of her mother's transgressions. Kucich notes both the tendency of Dickens's villains to be violent against themselves, citing Headstone's nosebleed, for example (73), and the tendency of his heroes to achieve integration through some scene of disintegration, whether of violence or of expenditure (108). Kucich's fine reading concentrates on a psychoanalytic vision of the self, but the key opposition he traces between excess and restraint, between disintegration and self-control, is one I will explore here in terms of the liberal vision of the individual and its relation to the social body. Dickens uses the individual body to stage the development of the good, self-contained subject.

Male characters in *Bleak House* convey their inadequate self-containment in what we have seen are conventional ways; Richard, addicted to Chancery, loses his suit and blood gushes from his mouth. Mr. Vholes, Richard's counselor, seems so self-contained as to be inhuman, but his greed is emblematized by his vampiric consumption of Richard (due to dyspepsia, he is unable, like Stoker's later vampire, to eat ordinary food). Mr. Krook, also greedy and obsessive, is, as is typical of mid-Victorian fiction's inappropriate working-class male, an alcoholic, and in Dickens's most dramatic illustration of a failure in self-control, he spontaneously combusts, coating the entire vicinity with a thick, greasy effluvium. Krook, the parodic other "Lord Chancellor," is made to stand in for the corrupt body politic in a thinly veiled allegory of revolution, and in rhetoric mirroring that used to describe the martyrdom of Jo ("dead . . . and dying around us thus every day"): "The Lord Chancellor . . . has died the death . . . of all authorities in all places under all names soever, where false pretences are made, and where injustice is done . . . it is the same death eternally—inborn, inbred, engendered in the corrupted humours of the vicious body itself, and that only—Spontaneous Combustion, and none other of all the deaths that can be died" (479).

It is bad government that causes such lack of control in its subjects. Richard's obsession is attributed by Jarndyce to Chancery: "It is in the subtle poison of such abuses to breed such diseases. His blood is infected, and objects lose their natural aspects in his sight" (517). It is, of course, also the suit that causes the contested property of Tom-All-Alone's to become the slum that it is, which in turn infects Esther: "There is not a drop of Tom's polluted blood but propagates infection and contagion somewhere. There is not an Atom of Tom's slime . . . but shall work its retribution, through every order of society" (654). The sanitary rhetoric identifies all of these deaths as extending from the same mismanagement of the body, political, social, and individual. The body that is "vicious," not self-contained but self-seeking and overly desirous, engenders in its own humors "the only death" possible—a death that ruptures and makes meaningless the boundaries of the body that should protect the subject's interiority (479).

Lady Dedlock, for example, having lost her character as a result of an early affair, famously proceeds rapidly to literalize her loss of identity by changing clothes with the brickmaker's wife. Since Lady Dedlock's identity is not "really" based on the truth of her subjectivity but on performance, especially on the props of class identity seen in her portrait in the Galaxy Gallery of British Beauty, she is unrecognizable when not clothed as Sir Leicester's wife. Police Inspector Mr. Bucket and Esther drive by her, seeing her body without seeing *her*.[2] She aims to commit suicide like her erstwhile lover, who has effaced his identity much more successfully—as a man, he can become Nemo, or no-man, whereas as a woman, she is liable to become anywoman, that is, subsumed in the mass of women, misidentified rather than simply deprived of the identity she never legitimately held in the first place. Like Mr. Dolls in *Our Mutual Friend,* she is assimilated to the muck of the street by the filthy graveyard from which emanates the fever that has disfigured Esther:

2. Note that Mr. Bucket, as a manager of criminal behavior, is suggestively named as a container of fluids.

"A thick humidity broke out like a disease. . . . Drenched in the fearful wet of such a place, which oozed and splashed down everywhere, I saw, with a cry of pity and horror, a woman lying—Jenny, the mother of the dead child" (844). But it is the mother of a living child—a child only thought dead—that Esther actually sees but cannot at first identify: "I . . . put the long dank hair aside, and turned the face. And it was my mother, cold and dead" (847).

The contaminated wetness of London breeds disease and confusion. The celebrated fog with which *Bleak House* opens is compared to Chancery, an institution that substitutes endless verbosity and formality for any real engagement between individuals and that therefore, instead of conferring benefits on its clients like a good social institution, turns vampiric and sucks them dry, like Mr. Vholes. It moves between the inappropriate anality of Chancery and its equally inappropriate orality; like any bloodsucking parasite, it turns blood into excrement. The mugginess of Holborn is history with a vengeance, combining the prehistoric with the modern and trapping the urban dweller in its moist clutches: "It would not be wonderful to meet a Megalosaurus . . . waddling . . . up Holborn Hill. . . . Foot Passengers . . . in a general infection of ill temper . . . [lose] their foot-hold at street-corners, where tens of thousands of other foot passengers have been slipping and sliding since the day broke (if the day ever broke) adding new deposits to the crust upon crust of mud" (11). So begins the novel, in which history is presented in geological terms and humanity, unenlightened by the day of reason that, perhaps, has yet to break, is trapped in the muddy grip of undifferentiated darkness—in which an infection of ill temper is matched by the "pestilence" of "sin" in Temple Bar (12). The lack of individuality in the temple is represented by such inadequately differentiated names as Chizzle and Mizzle; this matches the lack of significant differences among the political ruling classes (Doodle, Foodle, etc., vs. Cuffy, Buffy, etc.) emblematized in the equally dank Chesney Wold in Lincolnshire, also soaking wet. Women's hazardous passions draw them also to moisture—Lady Dedlock dies a sodden death, and the dangerous Hortense memorializes her hatred for Lady Dedlock by walking barefoot through the wet grass at Chesney Wold—an action that the onlookers see as potentially suicidal. This rain, in short, is general all over England.

All this wetness implies a dangerous state of bodily incontinence, an unclean condition. But we need not look as far as elaborate interpretations of moisture as metaphor. F. S. Schwarzbach observes, "The mud [on Holborn Hill] is made up of dirt, rubbish (*dust* in English idiom), and raw sewage, ends up in the Thames and then oozes downstream to the Essex marshes. There it rots and festers, soon producing infectious effluvia that are blown by the raw East Wind back over the city. *This* is the stuff of the novel's dense fog. . . . Dickens is pointing to a literal economy of filth and disease" (95). I would also point out that Dickens's use of the metaphor of palimpsestic time, in which prehistoric London and "modern" London are simultaneously present, takes advantage of the common description of the existence of sanitary nuisances as the coexistence of barbarism within the heart of civilization. The scandal of filth in the heart of the modern city is an actual scandal, covered in the papers nearly daily, of the uncivilized, grotesque body persisting in the midst of civilization.

As Peter Stallybrass and Allon White have argued, the nineteenth-century city is organized around the binaries of filth/cleanliness and the constant fear of their transgression, or contamination, resultant from desire. This fear "was articulated above all through the 'body' of the city," which had to be surveyed to be controlled (136). By the mid-century this surveillance—equated with the essence of civilization—was institutionalized in the mechanisms of sanitary inspection and had entered both literary and visual culture, the latter principally in the form of sanitary maps. The sanitary movement responded to overcrowding and epidemic disease by emphasizing the dangers of filth. Accumulated waste that earlier had been perceived as an unpleasant but unavoidable reality of life in the city now seemed evidence of a vicious, even murderous, disregard for life. Bodily wastes were no longer simply by-products of the life process but animated and hostile filth that would, given the chance, attack the body itself. The body and its continence, which also modeled the boundaries of the middle-class individual self, could be preserved only through a careful policing of the abject and the closure of the boundaries of the body, through which contaminated or contaminating fluids should neither enter nor escape. By mid-century the "lower bodily strata" of both city and its inhabitants that Stallybrass and White describe being identified with both sewage and underclass behaviors was increasingly troped both as disease and as antimodernity, as health and modernity in turn came to be identified with a careful mapping and containment of the city's (and city dwellers') "guts."

Sanitary reformers sought, precisely, to control this body. Schwarzbach observes that Dickens "uses a language of social analysis and a model of social reform derived from the medical [sector]. . . . The ideological structure of the text depends significantly on the discourse and paradigm of contemporary medicine" (93). Yet he also argues that, while Dickens certainly implicates himself in the social control advocated by medical discourse, he is critical of it as well, pointing to Mr. Bucket's complicity with Chancery and that institution's evils (99) and suggesting that "the novel voices . . . [the] fear, that the methodology and ideology of reform in some sense merely reproduce and reinforce the social structures that sustain England's pathological condition" (100), using the bricklayer's resistance to Mrs. Pardiggle as support for this statement. It has also been suggested that Dickens seeks to heal the division between public and private in this novel. I would argue, however, that Dickens is not so critical of social reform here as he is of institutions and individuals who seek not to connect with other human beings but to pursue their own interests using institutionalized social work as a platform—that is, of those who blend public and private—as we shall see. In other words, Dickens's efforts to heal the public and private divide are really directed at healing the breach in that divide—he directs his efforts toward keeping the public and private more fully separate. The wants of the body, including the sanitary reform of the city and the medical relief of the poor, are to be a public matter, whereas tutelary social work is to be quite strictly private—an extension of the domestic circle of duty.

As in sanitary literature, descriptions of poverty emphasize filth and dampness. The condition of Tom-All-Alone's is exemplary of this, as is the brickmaker's hovel, where the gardens "grow nothing but stagnant pools," the room is "damp and offensive," the people are mud-stained, and the daughter of the house hopelessly "washes" items in "very dirty water" (120–21). The man of the house, who has "been drunk for three days," makes his famous speech to Mrs. Pardiggle regarding the value of her officious social work, as he points to the physical conditions in which his family lives: "Look at the water. Smell it! That's wot we drinks. How do you like it and what do you think of gin, instead! . . . [My place] is . . . nat'rally dirty, and it's nat'rally onwholesome, and we've had five dirty and onwholesome children, as is all dead infants, and so much the better" (121). He finishes by bragging that he has beaten his wife, and is stolidly unmoved by Mrs. Pardiggle's "mechanical way of taking possession of people" like a "moral Policeman" (122). Mrs. Pardiggle's self-aggrandizing and "mechanical" application of a professionalized and fairly abstract religious process in "regular rotation" is clearly deprecated by the narrator. However, what is set in opposition to it—Ada and Esther's natural sympathy for the bereaved mother that achieves a personal connection with her—is precisely what middle-class women's social work is modeled on in this period. Dickens does not denounce this work so much as he denounces professionalization. Yet Ada and Esther's intervention is, finally, no more materially useful to the family than Mrs. Pardiggle's.

As in Gaskell's novel, fluidity tends to represent potentially uncontrollable forces—often, in Dickens, the forces of a specifically grotesque and diseased body. The city is an "ocean," and its children—always the site of potential renewal in Dickens—are always in danger of drowning. Charley runs to work "and melt[s] into the city's strife and sound, like a dewdrop in the ocean" (233). Jarndyce, of course, saves Charley—he makes her a maid and educates her and her siblings. We see her at last safely married in St. Albans. But Jo, whose brief life is spent sweeping the filth from the road, eventually goes under, as we might expect of someone attempting such a herculean task as the sweeping of London. In a poignant tableau, Jo sits eating near Blackfriars bridge, looking at the cross atop St. Paul's: "one might suppose that sacred emblem to be, in his eyes, the crowning confusion of the great, confused city; so golden, so high up, so far out of his reach. There he sits, the sun going down, the river running fast, the crowd flowing by him in two streams—everything moving on to some purpose and some end—until he is stirred up, and told to 'move on' too" (290–91). But, of course, Jo has no particular purpose that keeps him abreast of the current, and so drowns. He returns to his slum in St. Giles (Tom-All-Alone's), situated on its "stagnant channel of mud" (657), clothed in "shapeless clothes . . . [that] look, in color and substance, like a bundle of rank leaves of swampy growth, that rotted long ago" (659), degenerating into the primeval mud of Holborn. Chancery and its environs are also figured as a water world. Law and Equity are "ships" and the Inns during the long vacation are "like tidal harbors at low water . . . where stranded proceedings . . . lie high and dry upon the ooze of the long vacation" (278).

The Thames, of course, represents both the source of all this moisture and its potential for renewal. But the Thames is dark and polluted, and Esther's search with Mr. Bucket for her lost mother takes place in a nightmare landscape of Stygian waters: "We rattled . . . through such a labyrinth of streets, that I soon lost all idea of where we were; except that we had crossed and recrossed the river, and still seemed to be traversing a low-lying, waterside, dense neighborhood of narrow thoroughfares, chequered by docks and basins. . . . At length we stopped at the corner of a little slimy turning, which the wind from the river, rushing up it, did not purify" (803). This is a corner of the river where bodies are dragged up, and Mr. Bucket seeks Lady Dedlock there. Esther hears the tide repeatedly "rush" toward her (804) and fantasizes that she sees her mother's face rising up out of it.

Mr. Bucket's constant peering into the "black pit" of the river, at the woman's corpse that has been dragged out, and at the homeless women who walk near it emphasizes the femininity of this moistness and its deathliness; those who have lost their identities melt into this undifferentiated moisture. It is no wonder Esther fears that it is coming to get her, and no wonder that she can never see the river again after that night "free of the impressions of that journey" near the "dreaded water" (804); even the imperturbable Mr. Bucket is shocked to see "how wet you are!" (834). If they do not find Lady Dedlock at the riverside, perhaps that is because the water has expanded to cover the entire land, blanketed with muddy, melting snow that destroys the definition of the city: "The sleet fell all that day unceasingly, a thick mist came on early, and it never rose or lightened for a moment. Such roads I had never seen. I sometimes feared we had missed the way, and got into the ploughed grounds, or the marshes" (816). The roads are "as if they were torn up by a waterwheel" (819).

But in Esther's case, the dunking is a salutary heroic descent into the underworld, enabling her to move, with a little illness, beyond her mother's tale. Esther's is a true liberal story of individualism. Unlike Jane Eyre, whose temper is affected by her early privations and whose quest for independence can be completed only by the discovery of a respectable identity and blood relations, Esther's essential goodness—her core self—is untouched by her childhood experiences. She is initially both individually troubled and socially disadvantaged by her lack of identity, but her identity, as her multifarious names indicate, is not so important as her character, which overcomes even Mrs. Woodcourt's Welsh family pride. As with Lady Dedlock, because Esther is a woman—and a bastard—her precise identity is not her own. However, because she is a woman, this matters far less than Esther's domesticity and capacity for self-control and self-sacrifice. It is through this capacity for self-containment that Esther secures her individuality and her right to a happy marriage, rather than in an identity that is socially given, and which Dickens decries as therefore inherently fragile.

Esther demonstrates this capacity by refusing to ask about her antecedents when Jarndyce offers her the chance to do so (although, unbeknownst to her, he knows little more than she). Nevertheless, despite her early and frequent demonstrations of self-control, a society so massively infected as the London Dickens depicts demands its sacrificial victim. Dickens chooses to emphasize his sanitary moral—that all society is connected in its vulnerability to the poor self-containment of a few—by making Esther, the representative of the social ideal, bear on her body the marks of the social body's infection. Her fever dream, in which she is a bead on a flaming necklace, has been read as showing her need to be separate from Lady Dedlock, who is often associated with jewelry, and this is certainly correct. But that string of beads is also a symbol of Dickens's principal theme—the social connectedness of all the characters in the novel—that Esther represents in herself and from which she must also achieve a certain level of separation: "my only prayer was to be taken off from the rest. . . . It was such inexplicable agony and misery to be a part of the dreadful thing!" As is often the case in the fiction of the period, illness symbolizes a time of development, when Esther "cross[es] . . . a dark lake" and must make sense of all of her varied experiences from childhood to adulthood that confusingly coexist in her visions, welding them into a unitary self, laboring up "colossal staircases." She emphasizes that she is retelling it as a social duty: "It may be that if we knew more of such strange afflictions, we might be able to better alleviate their intensity" (514). In telling her story, Esther suggests that the causes of her suffering are endemic to an imperfect society but, with study, may be allayed. Individuals may be better able to emerge from that connectedness that is common to humanity, but that need not be so painfully fluid; a healthy social body promotes the closure, separation, and containment of individual bodies and selves.

Esther is pleased by her disfigurement when she reflects that it lessens the chance of Lady Dedlock's secret being discovered; more to the point, her loss of beauty forces others to evaluate her on the basis of her character alone, as she is stripped of other attractions. The discovery allows Esther to examine her fears and abolish her guilt over her birth in an egalitarian vision of the enlightenment subject as a being without original sin: "I was as innocent of my birth, as a queen of hers" (543). After the death of her mother, Esther falls ill again, but the sickness is "mild," takes place offstage, and seems to exist only to complete her transition to a wholly Adamic state, which enables Jarndyce to invite Mrs. Woodcourt into his home to begin the evaluation of Esther that is to overturn Mrs. Woodcourt's prejudices—though we never see exactly how—against Esther's birth. History, for Esther, is what can be made to cease hurting.

On the other hand, he who is too individualized—which Dickens figures as being self-absorbed to the exclusion of social or domestic connection—is also a problem. Such a person is dangerously close to *lumpen* in having no communitarian identity. Dickens avoids demonizing the poor in this way, instead choosing the irresponsible gentleman for this role: Skimpole. Although a much more charming and polished "Child" than the laborers who are figured in this way by Gaskell, Skimpole's character is much the more frightening one—a middle-class gentleman who has chosen to be a child, rather than being simply trapped in that developmental stage and therefore without hope of remediation, because without desire for it. Characteristic of paupers, he has a large family he cannot support, and his daughters in turn have begun to marry early and have children they cannot support, either.

Jarndyce is unable to see Skimpole's true nature, but the domestic woman, properly instructed by the real moral policeman, Bucket, learns to evaluate such characters correctly.[3] Bucket, strikingly, distracts Esther from worrying

3. Lauren Goodlad's *Victorian Literature and the Victorian State* focuses on the question of liberal leadership—the pastoral leadership that would lead while simultaneously fostering individual and local

about her mother during their journey by instructing her in the art of home-making, which is how he repeatedly characterizes his giving her tips about the behavior of various criminals, "advice that your husband will find useful when you are happily married and have got a family about you." Among these useful tips is the following: "Whenever a person proclaims to you 'In worldly matters I am a child, . . . you have got that person's Number, and it is Number One'" (810). Contrast this to the brickmaker, who contentiously demands recognition as an adult, deriding Mrs. Pardiggle's inane religious tract as unsuitable for his age: "I'm not a babby. If you was to leave me a doll, I shouldn't nuss it" (121). The brickmaker, unattractive as he is, is more comprehensible, as a creature produced in part by his environment, than Skimpole's monstrous perversion of the "normal" bourgeois desire for financial independence and personal and social self-sufficiency. The crime is perhaps all the more heinous since Skimpole is trained as a doctor and presumably understands the workings of the social. In contrast to the heroic physician Alan Woodcourt, who goes out of his way to help the dying Jo, Skimpole recommends that Jarndyce put the sick child out in the street, as "there is a bad sort of fever about him," and subsequently he betrays the boy to Bucket for five pounds.

In the same way, Dickens condemns both women and men, but especially women, who place their self-aggrandizement above service to the community—in women's case, to their own families. Mrs. Jellyby and Mrs. Pardiggle are paradigmatic failed social activists and are associated with the feminist Miss Wisk (445), who is committed to Woman's mission against her tyrant Man. Religion comes in for a share of such blame, as in the case of the nameless woman whose "church was like a fancy fair" but whose home was a "filthy wilderness" (444). Esther, who is able to make a home even in the savage jungle of Mrs. Jellyby's house, is the good domestic woman, who is modestly unsure of her ability to do good social work, and she suggests that she should "render what kind services I could, to those immediately around me; and to try to let that circle of duty gradually and naturally expand itself" (117).

Here we have Hill's stipulation for a charity that begins at home and is an extension of family relationships rather than an intrusion into the public sphere, such as Mrs. Jellyby's letters to the press on behalf of Africans she has never seen. The good domestic home operates as the ideal throughout the

---

development of the qualities necessary to govern. As she points out, fear of massification, countering the individualism so prized and simultaneously feared by Victorian political thinkers, is a key feature of the discourses of this period (and our own). In her reading of *Bleak House,* she sees Inspector Bucket as a failed pastor precisely because he does not react with sympathy to the slum dwellers' endurance of miserable sanitary conditions. We therefore understand, she argues, that he is simply perpetuating the massification of the residuum. Bucket, then, as policeman, represents the failure of middle-class leadership to transcend the status quo.

novel, through the initial and well-known opposition between Chesney Wold and Bleak House to the final metastasization of Bleak House away from St. Albans to Yorkshire. Esther joins her homemaking mission to Alan Woodcourt's vocation as a parish doctor—a fine model of successful social work that caps Esther's career of domesticating everything she touches, including Caddy Woodcourt, Charley, and so on, with, of course, the indispensable masculine help of Jarndyce, whose money quietly makes everything possible and who never performs his charity institutionally but strictly personally.

But the transformation of lives within the "circle of duty," however impressively epic Dickens manages to make it in *Bleak House,* is as drops in the ocean of London, as we are reminded by the death of Jo and the misery of the brickmakers' wives and children. The move to Yorkshire, seems, finally, a defeat for a novel so dependent on London topography, doubling Mary Barton's escape with Jem to pastoral Canada. Private charity transforms a bleak house into a home, but the city's bleakness remains untouched. Dickens finally has nothing better to offer than the ever-more-perfect separation between domestic and public life, in which the public is hopelessly corrupt and the domestic offers a tenuous and limited salvation for those within a small "circle of duty."

Our Mutual Friend: Filthy Desires

Keeping these points in mind, then, we can see that in *Our Mutual Friend* the iconography of the individual and urban social body operates in much the same way. Liquidity, garbage, filth, and waste constantly threaten the incautiously un-self-contained body. Much has been made of the contents of the dustheaps and whether we are to take them as containing feces or not. Setting aside the historical question of their likely contents, we should look at the literary question of their representation. There seems to be little doubt that the dustheaps are waste and represent, at least allegorically, human waste—as well as a human preoccupation with harmful things of no real value. In the summer they allure "all manner of crawling, creeping, and buzzing creatures, attracted by the gold dust of the Golden Dustman" (209), and Silas is confirmed in his suspicions of the hidden wealth in the dust mounds when Boffin demands that he read and reread the biography of the miser Dancer, especially the chapter on "The Treasures . . . of a Dunghill" (481), though all the misers' biographies emphasize the filth they live in, according to Dickens. Much has been made of the anality and excremental obsession of *Our Mutual Friend* (see especially Michael Steig and Catherine Gallagher) and the fecal equation with paper money; I would like to suggest that both greed and the abjected material of the body represent its dependence on others and lack of closure, its susceptibility to the mass humanity of barbarism/anarchy, rather than the clean individualism and bodily closure of civilization/culture.

Addiction—and greed for money comes under this heading in *Our Mutual Friend*—is even more markedly portrayed as desire for physical dissolution, for the abject. In greed, as in any essentially unfulfillable desire, there is something vampiric, as Dickens marks when he has Mortimer casually mention that old Harmon had himself buried "with certain eccentric precautions and ceremonies against his coming to life" (15). The investors whose delirious addiction "as under the influence of henbane or opium" pumps up the empty bubble of the Veneering estate invite greedy, phantasmic corporations to "fatten on us" (114). We also see more straightforward representations of addiction. The unfortunate Mr. Dolls, whose very name is unknown—he takes his name from his daughter's occupation, continuing the gross reversal of both gender and familial roles that Dickens famously uses to indicate rot in the familial and social body—drinks himself into a shambling and animalistic state of utter dependency. His daughter warns him of his impending disintegration: "you'll shake to bits" (714), she says, and threatens to pay the dustman to carry him off in his cart (532). He finally does shake to bits—simply disintegrating into a mass of rags and rotten vegetables from which his dead body cannot readily be distinguished.

However, successful self-production is not merely located in the coherence of the body. Silas Wegg looks forward to the day he will "collect myself like a genteel person": instead of being "dispersed, a part of me here, and a part of me there." Venus promises not to sell Silas's leg bone to anyone else, since Silas says he has "a prospect of getting on in life and elevating myself by my own independent exertions." Indeed, he is able to purchase the bone, but since his "independent exertions" actually manifest themselves as blackmail, he is really a parasite rather than a productive, independent self. Silas's bone is still available only because it has an invisible twist that makes it impossible to fit against other bones, so Venus speculates that perhaps its only value would be "as a Monstrosity" (82). On the other hand, the officially nameless Sloppy, called so "from being found on a sloppy night" (201), cannot manage his body particularly well, but through loyalty and love he manages to create a workable self and has a chance for economic independence as a cabinetmaker by the end of the story.

As in *Bleak House,* addiction can also manifest as obsession, either monetary or sexual. Eugene, the upper-class gentleman who appears to have the correctly contained bourgeois body but who in actuality lacks self-control, cruelly lampoons Mr. Dolls, "fumigating him" with disinfectant on burning charcoal while he interrogates him about Lizzie's whereabouts (*Our Mutual Friend* 538). This marks Mr. Dolls as waste material to be disinfected; still, like those human flies drawn to the dust mounds, Eugene cannot leave the abject alone. Eugene expresses scorn for most of the lower-class characters surrounding him; it is he who names Mr. Dolls, he who calls Bradley Headstone "Schoolmaster," professing not to be interested in his name—in short, it is he who carelessly denies others their own individuality and despises their weaknesses. Eugene, however, has himself succumbed to a sexual obsession with Lizzie—and subsequently, a sadomasochistic obsession with Bradley Headstone (whose association with anal rape has been elegantly elaborated by Catherine Gallagher).

Bradley Headstone should have gone to sea, as the narrator intimates, where he might have had relief from the "wild energy" that has "heaved up" the "bottom of this raging sea" in his breast (396), but he never masters that watery and unpredictable element of his subjectivity, and in the end he literally drowns. Eugene is duly punished for his lack of self-containment, which leads him to have such a dangerous contact with Mr. Dolls, and whose death he indirectly causes. When he uses the information he has received to find Lizzie, he is himself beaten to a bloody and undifferentiated pulp by Headstone and then dumped, like so much sewage, in the river from which Lizzie literally rebirths him, an act that finally rewards her own sexual self-containment, demonstrated throughout the novel and emblematized by her mastery over the water, with middle-class status. She is, as Mortimer insists, a "lady."

In Dickens, as in Gaskell, the body of the fit citizen is represented as a body that achieves closure. The depiction of addiction or other uncontrolled desire (financial speculation, obsession) as a kind of leakage in the individual that unfits one for citizenship and sinks one in the mass has, itself, a history of entanglement with representations of political resistance. In the next chapter we will examine something of the history of that representation and see how Eliot uses it in her own analysis of the development of the enlightenment self and in her conscious revision of the tradition of Condition of England novels on the theme of the franchise.

9

FELIX HOLT

The Desiring Body in the Later Political Novel

> Good society, floated on gossamer wings of light irony, is of very expensive production, requiring nothing less than a wide and arduous national life condensed in unfragrant deafening factories. . . . This wide national life is based entirely on emphasis—the emphasis of want, which urges it into all the activities necessary for the maintenance of good society and light irony. . . . Under such circumstances there are many among its myriads of souls who have absolutely needed an emphatic belief. . . . Some have an emphatic belief in alcohol and seek their *ekstasis* or standing ground in gin.
>
> —George Eliot, *The Mill on the Floss*

George Eliot's *Felix Holt* is a self-consciously anachronistic novel: set in the time of the first reform but addressing the second; reaching back to the tradition of overtly political novels like Disraeli's and yet fully cognizant of the innovations, both political and aesthetic, of the intervening decades. Mediating between the gender politics of the 1860s narrative and the generic demands of the political novel, Victorian literature offers a number of common tropes in the description of the body, both individual and social, and the threat posed by inappropriate bodies, inappropriate subjects. Dependency on alcohol and drugs becomes a common symbol of such threats and is often tied to class violence. By the 1860s, also, as Brantlinger argues, "the idea of culture . . . became crucial as a measuring stick of fitness of the working-class for political responsibility" (*Spirit* 239). Here culture is vague, but it generally has to do with education and the arts. Certainly one sees this in Arnold and Eliot. It is this culture, and the social progress of temperance and economic self-control that is thought to go hand in hand with it, that is posed explicitly as not merely the better alternative to politics for the working classes but the preliminary stage through which the potential citizen must pass to someday be ready for the political and public sphere.

Insatiable Desire: Aspiration and Addiction

Contemporary discussions of addiction today are often situated between the conflicting vision of the addicts as subject to an illness, entrenched within a complex set of social relations that contributes to their plight, and addicts as weak-willed, criminal individuals with sole responsibility for their sins. Often the second definition is considered a holdover from earlier times, and this is certainly consonant with the dominant discourse on substance abuse in nineteenth-century Britain. However, what I would like to examine here is an alternative history, in which both abuse and addiction are used quite early in the period to indicate social problems. If mid-Victorian liberalism depended on the management of desire, then that management was attended by anxiety about the ability of the social body to satisfy and direct the desires it had created.

Early on, abuse and addiction are used in fiction to represent this anxiety. This is especially evident in the social problem novels of the late 1840s, which created a context for later literary representations, particularly in the 1860s, when the sensation novel would come to represent the antisocial dangers of desire gone awry in the domestic sphere. George Eliot's *Felix Holt* of 1866 is a political novel both timely, appearing on the eve of the passing of the Second Reform Bill, and peculiar, seemingly reviving a form more suited to an earlier time. However, the novel is in fact remarkably up to date, revising the form of the social problem novel and taking advantage of plot devices borrowed from the sensation novel—that degenerate parody of the hegemonic domestic narrative—to offer Eliot's take on the problematic of desire in capitalist culture. Taking up the topic of addiction from contemporary debates, Eliot uses it to argue that the mismanagement of desire is the central problem of liberal government, both in the public sphere of the social problem novel's cryptopolitical realm and the private, domestic sphere of the sensation novel. Self-consciously repeating the formula of earlier novelists so often reproached by critics[1]—dovetailing the social and economic narrative into one of individual courtship—she illustrates her sense that the two stories, and indeed the preoccupations of very different genres more than a decade apart, are two sides of the same coin.

The sensation novel craze in the 1860s was, as many critics have noted, constructed by contemporary critics around anxieties about women's voracious appetites for certain kinds of information and certain kinds of narratives, an appetite that was often compared to addiction and narratives that

1. Most famously, Raymond Williams.

were often compared to drugs and alcohol.[2] Both in this discourse and within the literature itself, we see dramatizations of addiction as a model of inappropriate desire that undermines citizenship and the social body. However, addiction is precisely so appropriate a model because it highlights the inherent danger of using capitalism to mobilize social and political compliance. It is the nature of (especially commodity) capitalism to create desire that quickly becomes need, which generates more desire. It is its nature, in other words, to create *unfulfillable* desires. The desire for upward mobility that was to act as a disciplinary construct is, in fact, one of those desires. As in addiction, the very gratification of the desire leads to a tendency to exceed the individual's ability to gratify it as a need—a model of immoderate need that leads inevitably to loss, to the destruction of the body, individual and social. If the model of the social body worked out in this period depended upon the inculcation and management of individual desires, then addiction represents anxiety about the systemic inability of the social body to contain the desire that it has created.

In the early to mid-nineteenth century the connection of the individual to the social body is articulated through the capitalist economy and is elaborated in terms of desire—biological desire leading to reproduction giving rise to economic desire leading to production. Appropriate behavior is inculcated through domesticity, which inspires the desire for upward economic mobility—husbands wish to house their wives, parents desire respectability and economic security for their young children and then develop class ambitions for them as adults in turn seeking marriage and career. These desires act as guarantees of good economic and social behavior—the worker will be law abiding, hardworking, and temperate, the homemaker prudent and thrifty. As Bentham remarked, "A wife and children are so many pledges a man gives to the world for his good behavior" (*Principles* 174n1).

As we have seen, however, a large class, often conceptualized under the rubric of pauperism, posed a problem for the social body and its modes of control mapped by capitalism. Paupers had two problems: too much biological desire and not enough social desire, leading to reproduction without forming heterosexual patriarchal families and thus without economic desire or production. Paupers were by definition people who did not want to be upwardly mobile—at least, not as Victorian social theorists understood upward mobility. This group, however, did not account for two other classes of individuals, related to but not exactly coterminous with paupers. The first group comprised those whose economic ambitions were not linked to repro-

2. See Kate Flint, *The Woman Reader*, and Gilbert, *Disease, Desire and the Body*.

ductive familial respectability—criminals, frauds, and so forth. Set apart by their unusual lack of connection to the social body, these might, for the most part, be dealt with as aberrations. The second group, far more problematic, is that of individuals who, having internalized all the desires and behaviors of proper bourgeois social life, were still unable to follow out that path of social development. Again, these cases tend to be treated as aberrations in literature outside of the social problem novel. But when such individuals were read as representative of a class, as they were in social problem fiction arising out of the economic reversals of the hungry 1840s—persons whose desire, being thwarted, might assume monstrous proportions or be unsatisfiable—then they become representative of revolutionary fears signaled by a desire without moderation, a hunger that does not die. This hunger, troped as vampirism in analyses of capitalism and desire by authors as diverse as Marx (*Das Kapital*) and Dickens (Vholes in *Bleak House*), is also associated with addiction and drugs, alcohol, and gambling, especially earlier in the century.

Middle-class women and the working classes generally were the two groups most commonly associated with the habitual use of drugs in this period.[3] Most historians correctly point out that our constructions of addiction and its connections to socioeconomic problems cannot be neatly projected onto the early nineteenth century. Outside of a few notable authors such as Thomas De Quincey, who does not see his addiction either as a disgrace or as a social problem, addiction is largely ignored by creative writers.[4] Although Victorian drunkenness is frequently a topic of interest among scholars, as recently as 1996 Josephine Guy argued that it was perceived not as a social problem but one of individual self-control. Until recently, opium and other intoxicant addictions were generally thought not to be a topic of public debate at all until the 1860s;[5] Geoffrey Harding and Barry Milligan have done much to dispel this oversimplified view. Harding remarks on the significant attention

3. See Stephen Kandall, for example.

4. See, for example, Terry Parsinnen: "[Opium addiction] was for the most part, a nonissue. Medical men wrote about it rarely; popular writers almost never. And when people thought about it at all, they thought that addiction was a relatively infrequent, if unfortunate, by-product of the therapeutic use of an important drug."

5. Parsinnen states that Victorians were not concerned about the dangers of opiates until the 1870s but admits that the Poisons and Pharmacy Act was passed in 1868. Certainly, the Victorians were agitated a good deal about opium in the 1860s, as evidenced by a slew of publications, including *The Mystery of Edwin Drood*, and by the Poisons and Pharmacy Act itself. Interestingly, the only attention given to opium as an *addictive* drug is through the focus on opium smoking, associated with the Chinese, which scholars now agree was quite rare among the English, most of whom preferred their opium in stronger forms, available for a penny at the local pharmacy.

paid to opium use among the working class and concern over the "doping" of infants in the 1840s (13–15). Milligan finds evidence of concern even earlier, noting that as early as the 1816 publication of *Kubla Khan,* there was anxiety about the abuse of opium by the uneducated working classes. Still, he indicates that generally this was seen in the light of a failure in individual will and also that working-class use was seen as "chronic intemperance" rather than addiction.

Although I would agree that this is most often the case, I would like to argue that a significant number of social narratives do early on recognize a cultural component in "setting the stage" for at least the abuse of drink or opium. Here it is necessary to clarify some terms. "Addiction," with the medical and legal meanings we have come to associate with it, is indeed largely a twentieth-century construct. Very often, working-class habitual use of drink or drugs is represented as simple abuse and not addiction. However, many authors do describe the use of both drink and opium as a habit that comes to master its users, changing their behavior and subordinating it to the need for the substance. It is this second type of representation that I am here terming addiction. Both abuse and addiction, however, may be used by Victorians as indices of social distress and thwarted desire, and it is this usage I am concerned with here. For example, in sanitary narratives the uncleanliness of the home is often blamed for working men's drinking. While the working-class wife is often the target of culpatory gestures in such texts, many sanitarians point to the physical conditions of poor neighborhoods in frustrating the wife's efforts to create an appropriately domestic space, thus describing a vicious cycle—a bad neighborhood undermines the wife's efforts, which prompts the husband's drinking out of desire for comfort, which results in counterproductive economic behavior, trapping the family in a downward spiral in which they move to progressively worse neighborhoods. In short, while those narratives that blame individuals for drinking castigate them for not having appropriate desires, those that situate such behavior in a social cause identify the drinking worker as the bearer of a desire perverted by social conditions that undermine the natural domesticity that would foster desire's appropriate investments.

Given these points, it is perhaps not surprising that drinking and drug taking are inscribed not only as individual failures but less frequently, though still importantly, as failures in social control. These behaviors can be scripted as indictments of a system that inculcates desires that not only cannot be fulfilled but cannot even be appropriately pursued. For the point of such desire is not to fulfill it—with commodity capitalism, there is no fulfillment, only limitless movements of desire spiraling upward—but to gratify it continuously just enough to control its track. Thus, cravings for drink and drugs come to model not only desire gone wrong but also efforts at social control by a bourgeois elite who cannot manage the desire they have created in a proletariat "brought in from the cold" of pauperism to an even colder and hungrier respectable poverty.

Thus, by the 1860s one has Marx's remark that "religion is the opium of the people"—self-medication, certainly, but with a patent medicine sold by and profited from by an elite who manufactured Godfrey's cordial by the barrel and Christian tracts by the ream. In short, habitual use of or addiction to alcohol or drugs was seen quite early on as a working-class response to dissatisfaction with society's inability to feed appetites that were considered appropriate and necessary—which it had even deliberately fostered. In this context, many writers perceived—and critiqued—the potential use of drugs to control the working class and subvert aggression or revolution (after all, this was a country that immediately saw the potential of addicting Chinese consumers in order to control the balance of trade). However, at the same time, drugs and alcohol clearly represented desire possibly *out* of control—the kind of frustration that could end in a drunken riot, for example, and the destruction of life and property. Therefore, representations of addiction or drug abuse sometimes indicate a failure of will or individual morality but often also an indictment of society's inadequacies and, at other times still, elite attempts to control a population whose legitimate desires cannot be met, by preventive medication.

Attention to the "problem" elements of the social body (at different times identified as paupers, unionists, transgressive women, etc.) by the late 1840s highlighted individuals who, having internalized all the desires and behaviors of proper bourgeois social life, were still unable to follow out that path of social development. Kingsley's *Alton Locke* is a teetotaler who watches the tailors around him drink themselves into poverty and death, to the destructions of the families that should have kept them sober and thrifty but could not because they were unsupported by the economic structure (one man watches his wife and children die and be eaten by rats while he suffers from delirium tremens). Locke is a clear precursor to Shaw's Major Barbara, who cries in despair that Bodger's whiskey is her greatest enemy in saving the people of the East End. While riding through the fens area of England, Locke is horrified to learn of the "penny a day of comfort" opium habits of the inhabitants (the fens area produced its own opium). The madness for drink in *Alton Locke* is tied to the "sweating" system of exploitation of the workers—the only alternative, however, for the workers who cannot escape the system is Chartism and revolution. In the countryside, furious and starving workers riot and steal alcohol. The resulting drunkenness carries the crowd into arson. In *Mary Barton* Gaskell's John Barton is driven by hunger and rage at the masters to take opium, to which he becomes addicted to the point that he finally prefers it to food. (We see here the logic of the substitute that comes to take precedence over the original, healthy desire.) His domestic life has been destroyed, first by the starvation of his son and later, after rebuilding, by his loss of work. One by one, his household items are sold off, and the hearth, symbol of domestic comfort, is cold for lack of fuel; nevertheless, he sits there "(from habit), smoking or chewing opium . . . strange faces of pale men, with dark glaring eyes . . . beckoned him away. . . . They were all desperate members of trades' unions, ready for any thing; made ready by want" (136). It is in this unhealthy state that Barton shoots Harry Carson, the master's son. From the description of the union meeting, Gaskell shifts immediately to a discussion of how factory work for women makes them unfit wives, unable to prepare edible food, and then, again, immediately to John Barton's encounter with Esther, the prostitute.

In this novel, Barton's opiate abuse is thematically and structurally connected both to union agitation and violence and to the prostitution of Esther, Mary's aunt, whose immoderate class ambition leads to extramarital sexual desire. Infatuated with "one above me far," she is seduced and abandoned with a baby daughter. Forced into prostitution to get medicine for her ailing infant in a cruel parody of the economic aspirations of the legitimate family, she is driven, finally, to drink to escape both her grief when the child dies and her shame for her own disgrace. Fully addicted, she refuses to be saved from the streets because she cannot face the pains of withdrawal and the visions she suffers in the delirium tremens. The woman's immoderate desire and sexual transgression are connected to the worker's revolutionary violence through the destruction of the domestic sphere, from which desire can "normally" be appropriately directed. But the domestic sphere itself is destroyed by the capitalism that constitutes it and dictates its uses—the need of the cotton mills to remain competitive. The use of unsatisfiable hungers to symbolize society's failure to make good on its promises continues through the 1850s—as in *Bleak House* and the chancery suitors who, emaciated and unnaturally excited, are clearly addicted to Chancery itself, or Headstone's obsession with Eugene in *Our Mutual Friend,* who effortlessly incorporates the class habitus Headstone has worked so hard for but failed to fully acquire.

Addiction, Genre, and Desire: *Felix Holt* Rewrites the Condition of England Novel

In the 1860s discussion of the social issues of citizenship and representation called up by the Second Reform Bill shared newspaper space with the dangers to British identity posed by orientalized opium addiction. The decade also sees the blossoming of the sensation novel, famously preoccupied with consumption, class ambition, and transgressive female sexuality. Although there is still concern about the habits of the working class, in the wake of divorce reform and increasing women's activity outside the home, it is women's desires that come to preoccupy British readers. In M. E. Braddon's *Lady Audley's Secret,* Lady Audley's appetites for material goods and upward mobility lead her to separate herself from her child and attempt the murder of her first husband; her nerves require liberal applications of drugs, and, in her worst moment, she considers ingesting a suicidal dose of opium before simply self-medicating with laudanum instead. Her separation from her child and even her earlier class ambition is in turn fostered by her father's alcoholism and consequent indebtedness.[6]

Discussions of sensation novels externalized their thematizations of vampiric materialism by describing the novels themselves as drugs or drams and readers as addicted "lotus-eaters" whose healthy appetites were thus being destroyed, replaced by inappropriate ones. Working-class readers, also, were singled out for surveillance—what was to stop them from enacting these fictional hungers themselves, working women from attempting to seduce wealthy men into marriage and impressionable working-class boys from imitating the highwayman heroes of penny dreadfuls? The sudden fascination with Chinese opium dens, exemplified in *The Mystery of Edwin Drood,* emerges out of a xenophobic orientalism in which opium represents social control by an external agent rather than an internal one—British readers fascinated and horrified by the spectacle of a few female British opium smokers consorting with Chinese men conveniently forgot the vast quantities of opium orally ingested in practically every British household. As Milligan points out, engrossed with fears of racial degeneration and "infection" by Eastern elements, Britain projects her own guilty history during the opium wars—the deliberate attempt to addict Chinese to British-grown Indian opium in order to balance the trade deficit—onto a pipe-wielding Chinese counterinvasion. In this case the appetites mobilized for internal social control and the health of the social body are

6. Even her precocious child, Georgy, demonstrates the corrupting influence of his elders on his appetites by his refusal of children's food and insistence on "something savoury" with ale (179).

susceptible to foreign takeover. These desires can be redirected to the biting hungers and dreamlike satisfactions of the dockland dens, invading clean and proper British society through the orientalized English woman.[7]

From the social problem novel that monitors addiction, to the sensation novel, the mass culture commodity that mimics and symbolizes its pleasures, the discourse on addiction is tied to capitalism and its discontents in the control of the social body. I would like to turn now to the less obvious adumbration of this theme in a novel that has not been discussed in this context, George Eliot's *Felix Holt, the Radical.* Reacting to some extent against the sensation novel, Eliot writes a realist novel in which her usual themes (and indeed, the temporal setting of *Middlemarch* and *Mill on the Floss*), and especially those she later explored in *Daniel Deronda* (addiction and gambling as emblematic of other immoderate hungers, etc.), are examined in the context of elections following the first Reform Bill of 1832. *Felix Holt* was written while the second Reform Bill was being discussed and published a year before it passed; indeed, after it passed, Eliot famously was solicited to and did write an address to the working man on his new responsibilities as voter in the persona of Felix himself. Some have discussed the orientalist features of the novel and Eliot's destabilization of national and racial boundaries. But the connection between Eliot's exploration of imperial identity and her treatment of immoderate desire—most obviously embodied by the adulterous Mrs. Transome and the bastard Harold—has been neglected by critics. The thematics of addiction in the novel bind it to both the sensation novel and the social problem novel and illustrate the continuities in the treatment of addiction that I have outlined thus far. Eliot rewrites the late 1840s social problem novel and uses 1860s sensational plot elements to connect the preoccupation of contemporary citizenship debates—the appropriate management of desire, figured as drug-taking behaviors—to contemporary concerns about sexual and political transgression.

Kathleen McCormack observes that Eliot is particularly heavily invested in the drug metaphor for writing, throughout her career.[8] This is hardly

7. In *The Moonstone*, a more blatant "oriental revenge" story, William Wilkie Collins narrates how British imperial greed leads to the theft of the Indian sacred stone that brings danger to the innocent British woman. Shenanigans with opiates are the source of the mystery that nearly undoes the protagonists—in the end it takes an opium-addicted Eurasian to unravel the mystery. As Milligan points out, both Blake and Jennings (the Eurasian) in this story are cultural hybrids resulting from imperialism, and this hybrid nature makes them susceptible to opium.

8. I am working here from McCormack's article "George Eliot and the Pharmakon." For a discussion of drugs and their relation to the diseased social body throughout Eliot's work, see

surprising given the prevalence of that metaphor throughout the period, especially in critical reviewing. However, Eliot's use of this metaphor was more than accidental. McCormack observes that Eliot's notebooks reveal a fascination with the workings of drugs, particularly opium, and that she had very decided opinions about drugs and their relationship to patients' abilities to uphold social duties: "the novels . . . overtly support her statement in an 1860 letter . . . that doing one's duty as a Victorian demands going without opium, a stance all the more heroic for a perennial invalid" (39). McCormack demonstrates that Eliot was reading a good deal about opium in the 1860s and was particularly fascinated with opium's ability to have opposite effects depending on what drugs it was combined with and the state of the system it entered. McCormack is interested in the way Eliot uses drugs in her novels to "manifest power . . . at the same time they represent the power of the written word to remedy or aggravate the [political] ills of society"—if used responsibly—or to be damaging if used irresponsibly (40). This analysis is particularly useful in that it highlights Eliot's awareness of the (at least) dual potential of substances that is best captured in our own day by the dichotomy of meaning implied in the pair "medicine/drug." I would like to link McCormack's insight to the dual understanding of drugs in the Victorian period, as the model of social control through desire becomes problematized through the metaphor of addiction, and to examine how Eliot's discussion of addiction, inappropriate desire, and national identity both corresponds to and revises existing discourses.

Felix Holt has many drug-taking and drug-dispensing characters, and some who fit both categories. As McCormack points out, both "Mrs. Holt and Mrs. Transome dispense medicines indiscriminately, Christian takes opium recreationally, and Harold Transome and his cohorts treat with alcohol the uneducated patrons of the local ale houses whose condition Felix seeks to improve" (41). As McCormack also observes, dispensing drugs is itself "the opiate of her [Mrs. Transome's] discontent" (42). This introduces an unusual twist—a character whose addiction is to medicating others. The protagonist Felix Holt, however, fights to close the successful business he has inherited, selling worthless patent medicine, because as a trained apothecary he knows the medicine is valueless. The ability to "drug" others in this novel represents social power, just as Felix's desire to substitute meaningful progressive rhetoric and sanitary advice for demagoguery and patent nostrums represents social responsibility. Materially well off but comfortless and powerless over her own fate, Mrs. Transome's addiction is to power, as Eliot makes clear: "what could

---

McCormack's *George Eliot and Intoxication.*

then sweeten the days to a hungry, much exacting self like Mrs. Transome's? Under protracted ill every living creature will find something that makes a comparative ease, and even when life seems woven of pain, will convert the fainter pang into a desire. Mrs. Transome . . . found the opiate for her discontent in the exertion of her will about smaller things" (30). Throughout the novel, Eliot emphasizes that it is not just substances that are addictive but desire itself.

Eliot disliked sensation novels, yet she chose to use many sensational elements in *Felix Holt,* emphasizing the connection between the domestic realm of the women and the political arena in which the men predominantly figure. As in much sensation fiction of the time, the aristocratic woman has a sexual secret, and she is in effect blackmailed by a man who has the key to that secret. Early in her married life, she had an affair with her lawyer, by whom she has a son, now home from running a business in the Levant to claim the Transome estate. The lawyer, Jermyn, has had rather too free a hand with the family finances, largely because of his connection to Mrs. Transome. Mrs. Transome's illicit satisfactions, however, are not the origin of the breakdown of the Transome family, as they would be in most sensation novels. Her own transgression with Jermyn is rooted in frustration with the idiocy of her paralytic husband and his eldest born, who inherits his decadent body and the vicious mind, if not of his father, then of his grandfather ("even," as Eliot says, "to the third generation"). Mrs. Transome's appetite for Jermyn also stems from frustrated maternal desire. Indeed, when Jermyn's son Harold is born, she desires the death of her licit firstborn, so that Harold may inherit the wealth and name to which he bears no biological right. But the first son's idiocy itself is spawned out of inappropriate sexual desire on the part of a male Transome. In a move foreshadowing the 1890s indictment of syphilitic fathers, Eliot makes clear in her introductory chapter that the Transome degeneration is due to "some quickly satiated desire that survives, with the life in death of old paralytic vice, to see itself cursed by its woeful progeny" (10). This degeneration can also be seen in old Tommy Trounsem, the alcoholic last living Transome of his line.

Scorning conventional morality as "stupid and drug-like," fit only for the social control of inferiors, Mrs. Transome has no moral defenses against her own desires, which cannot be satisfied. Mrs. Transome, who is constantly described as "hungry" with "a void which could not be filled," had hoped her son would fill that void and

> give unity to her life . . . but the mother's early raptures had lasted but a short time, and even while they lasted there had grown up in the midst of them

> a hungry desire, like a black poisonous plant feeding in the sunlight,—the desire that her first . . . child should die. . . . Such desires make life a hideous lottery, where every day may turn up a blank; where men and women who have the softest beds and the most delicate eating, who have a very large share of that sky and earth which some are born to have no more of than the fraction to be got in a crowded entry, yet grow haggard, fevered and restless, like those who watch in other lotteries. (23)

As is here implied, Mrs. Transome's affair with Jermyn and even maternity of Harold take the place of opiates; they pretend to sate but actually create new desire.

In addition to the discontented upper-class woman, here both addicted and adulterous, *Felix Holt* shows the usual Condition of England novel's attention to working-class abuses of drink and makes the usual link with violence and revolution. It is particularly important that, in the wake of the Second Reform Bill, it is precisely the class left disenfranchised by the first bill that riots in the novel's 1833 setting—a class that is part of Eliot's newly enfranchised readership in 1867. Felix, who sees drink as the worst enemy of his attempts to educate the workers, protests the electioneering "treating" of workers who cannot vote but are used to intimidate the opposition. Jermyn and Johnson, election agents, protest that giving alcoholic bribes is required to manage the voting event. Johnson also explains that in order to motivate voters, it is necessary to mobilize the women: "one fourth of the men never would have voted if their wives hadn't driven them to it for the good of their families" (188).

Here we see the split persistently illustrated in this literature—those who have some potentially profitable investment in the social body are to be managed through their familial investments, and those outside must be managed with intoxicants—a dicey business since the intoxicants given to manage their behavior may eventually serve to make them unmanageable. This is a typical theme of the 1840s novel, but Eliot uses it to her own ends in the context of the second Reform Bill. In her "Address to the Working Men, by Felix Holt" Felix suggests that most working men are intemperate, wasting "on their own drinking the money that should have helped to feed and clothe their wives and children," and asks, "Where would be the political power of the thirty sober men [out of one hundred typical working-class votes]? The power would lie with the seventy drunken and stupid votes" (294). But who is supplying the drink? Of course, once the nonvoting laborers are made drunk by the "radical" candidate Harold's treating, they riot and attempt murder on the day of the election.

However, the avoidance of desire is not Eliot's answer, either. After an initial period of debauchery, Felix attempts to avoid even socially sanctioned desire: "he evaded calamity by choosing privation" (356), preferring to live on turnips rather than be tempted by sexual desire into marriage, which he believes must inevitably compromise his principles by forcing him to meet the needs of a wife and children. Felix's radicalism initially appears to be assisted by this principled rejection of social investments that imply social constraints; as Jermyn muses, he is "a young man with so little of the ordinary Christian motives as to making an appearance and getting on in the world, that he presented no handle to any judicious and respectable person who might be willing to make use of him" (185). He is willing to live frugally to the point of asceticism. Felix refuses to sell the patent medicines upon which his father built his modest fortune, because, as he has studied medicine, he knows their dangers: "'My father was ignorant . . . he knew neither the complication of the human system, nor the ways in which drugs counteract each other'" (61).

Eliot persistently connects addiction to both capitalism and social control.[9] As a radical who wishes for a true liberation of the people, which depends on weaning them off intoxicating drugs and false promises, Felix represents a threat both to the status quo and to the commercial ethos on which it is based. When Felix is arrested, mistakenly believed to have led the riot, Mrs. Holt sees it as a judgment: "he had put a stop to the making of saleable drugs, contrary to the nature of buying and selling" (352). After all, she says later, "what folks can never have boxes enough of to swallow, I should think you have a right to sell" (415). But what Felix wants to persuade the workers to take is exactly the bitter medicine that most do not want to "swallow," it being a painfully acquired taste.

However, Felix must be brought by the end of the novel to acknowledge his desire for Esther and renounce his renunciation of domesticity and paternity. Temperance and self-control are achieved not through the avoidance of temptation and desire but through daily struggle and compromise. But as is usual with Eliot, the principal problems of desire are situated in the woman

9. Mr. Christian, the butler, falls asleep on a stump after taking opium. He takes opium not only to relieve pain but to mask it: "Next to the pain itself he disliked that anyone should know of it; defective health diminished a man's market value." However, "certain conditions of his system had determined a stronger effect than usual" (143), and he passes out. This sets off the chain of events that results in the identification of Esther as the heir to the Transome estate. Christian's addiction—and it is defined by the narrator as a need for increasing dosages that will one day end in suicide—is linked in part to his ethically weak character. Still, here Eliot clarifies that there may be economic reasons for a worker's addictive behavior.

poised on the brink of adulthood. Through Esther, as she will later do with Maggie Tulliver and Gwendolen Harleth, Eliot points out clearly that the same desire that leads to spiritual growth leads to addiction; the problem is in channeling it. Esther's "hunger" for higher things, initially and harmfully focused on material objects, later becomes focused on spiritual development and Felix. Her hunger, therefore, is the basis of both her goodness and her temptation: "it comes in so many forms in this life of ours—the knowledge that there is something sweetest and noblest of which we despair, and the sense of something present that solicits us with an immediate and easy indulgence" (406)—which, in this case, is Harold's courtship. When she tells him playfully that she only likes what she cannot have, he offers her a superficially respectable temperance in answer:

> "I am very fond of things that I can get. And I never longed much for anything out of my reach. Whatever I feel sure of getting, I like all the better. I think half those priggish maxims about human nature in the lump are no more to be relied on than universal remedies. . . . Some are given to discontent and longing, others to securing and enjoying. And let me tell you, the discontented longing style is unpleasant to live with." (410).

Offering her the drug of an easy material well-being, he requires that she give up that hunger that makes her, for Eliot, most fully human.

Hitherto, Eliot suggests, this natural human desire for "higher things" has been a force that political economists have attempted to manage, without respect for the humanity and multifarious desires of individuals, and therefore without success: "Fancy what a game chess would be if all the chessmen had passions and intellects, more or less small and cunning. . . . You might be the longest headed of deductive reasoners, and yet you might be beaten by your own pawns. You would be especially likely to be beaten, if you depended arrogantly on your mathematical imagination, and regarded your passionate pieces with contempt" (278). Eliot is speaking of Jermyn here, but the quintessential political economist in the novel is Harold, the advocate of "an active industrious selfishness" he associates with the East (183), who thinks of servants as machines. Self-interest is a fragile concept on which to found a system of government, Eliot suggests. But even when it works, this "middle way" of temperance out of self-interest ultimately may be even worse than unrestrained gratification, which at least ultimately disgusts—as Felix's few weeks of debauchery make an abstainer out of him—or absolute asceticism, which is unrealistic. The successful capitalist, gaining his rewards out of enlightened self-interest, may superficially appear to be a fine citizen, but real citizenship, for Eliot, involves cultivating in oneself and others a hunger for higher goals than material improvement.

Harold, who "never forget[s] places and people—how they look and what can be done with them," whose native land lies "like a map on [his] . . . brain" (22) as though he has come to conquer it rather than to reintegrate himself into its communities, is the very type of both capitalist and imperialist. Opposed to Felix as part of the second mother-son pair and the other "radical" of the novel, he belies his radicalism with his imperious ways, which include both slave ownership and his operatives' willingness to dose the working population with drink to win the election, in contrast to Felix's refusal to drug them with patent concoctions. A self-defined "oriental" (194) who smokes a "hookah" (196) and is particular about his sauces, Harold also ironically embodies another late 1860s obsession, the East invading the West and enslaving Britons to opium. Eliot constructs Harold's history in such a way that readers are enabled to see him as an opium dealer. Not only does this complement Felix's role as trained apothecary refusing to drug the masses, but it also provides an ironic rereading, by Eliot, of the prevailing stereotype of the Chinese drug seller. The theme of the upstart bourgeois made rich on questionable foreign enterprise, returning to campaign against the landed family, is a common one, and the identification of the drug trade with suspicious politics has precedent in the reform novel. Disraeli pits "A Scotchman, richer than Croesus, one McDruggy, fresh from Canton, with a million of opium in each pocket, denouncing corruption and bellowing free trade" against his Young England hero Egremont (*Sybil* 70).

Terry Parsinnen notes that "most of the opium that was consumed in nineteenth-century Britain was grown in Turkey. . . . It could be cheaply produced by Turkish peasants; and its production was centralized around the Anatolian town of Afiun ('opium' in Turkish), only fifty miles inland from the port of Smyrna" (11).[10] He observes that "British firms, based in Smyrna, controlled virtually the entire trade in opium until the later nineteenth century, when they began to be challenged by Americans" (14). He adds, "In addition to the size of the crop, the opium trade was influenced by speculators at three key points in the market chain: in the Anatolian interior, where the crop was purchased from Turkish peasants by Greek and Armenian merchants who often kept them in debt-slavery; in Smyrna, where European drug traders purchased the opium from merchants; and in London, where wholesale

10. According to Parsinnen, Turkey became the fourth largest export market for Britain by the mid-century and sold various agricultural products to Britain, including corn (the largest export at, in 1860, 825,000 pounds sterling), along with a number of other products, including opium (187,000 pounds sterling in the same year).

drug dealers . . . bought opium at auction" (15).

Eliot, then reading material on opium wherein its geopolitical origins were quite clear, gives Harold the following history: instead of becoming a British diplomat, as was intended, "he had saved the life of an Armenian banker, who in gratitude had offered him a prospect which his practical mind had preferred to the problematic promises of diplomacy and high-born cousinship. Harold had become a merchant and a banker at Smyrna" (24). Eliot systematically gives Harold geographic and economic associations with the British pharmaceutical opium trade, thus balancing him ironically against Felix, her other radical and pharmaceutical businessman. In the context of Eliot's ongoing interest in the dangers of drugs, and especially opium, during the writing of this novel (which Kathleen MacCormack ably documents), her construction of his character both takes advantage of contemporary fears and fantasies about "orientals" and provides a corrective—the real drug peddler is a respectable British businessman in Smyrna, not a Chinese docklands den master. (Even his courtship of Esther is figured as a dangerous drug.) As with his electioneering agents, his status as merchant keeps his hands literally clean of the trade that Felix, who would actually handle drugs, rejects, but they are two extremes of the same industry process—a process that, Eliot reminds us, depends on slavery, tyranny, and all that 1860s debate in England aims to denounce. The Giaour who should rescue the Oriental woman instead enslaves her for his own use; Esther's Byronic fantasies are violently rewritten.

Harold's attitude to the domesticity that is the heart of the social order is telling. Uninterested in an English wife, who "would want to give [her] . . . opinion about everything" (20), he prefers the harem image of the oriental woman: "Western women were not to his taste: they showed a transition from the feebly animal to the thinking being, which was simply troublesome. Harold preferred a slow-witted, large-eyed woman, silent and affectionate, with a load of black hair weighing much more heavily than her brains. He had seen no such woman in England, save one he had brought with him from the East" (344–45). Outside of this surprising reference, this woman is never seen, and given that little Harry's mother is dead, it seems that the implication is that this woman is kept on the side as Harold courts Esther. Harold has actualized his harem.

Barry Milligan observes that by the 1860s writers on the opium dens not only exoticized them as oriental but also "portray[ed] Englishwomen assimilated—by both opium addiction and sexual unions with Chinese opium masters—to opium dens and Oriental identities" (13). Milligan also observes that the "reverse market control" symbolized by the Chinese den master's power over his customers dramatizes the instability of "market driven aspects of the power-dynamics of empire" (13). The second opium war of 1860 fueled public awareness of the British role in addicting Chinese (ibid., 27). Milligan notes the complex gender dynamic of the Orient as both the raped and the rapist, the infecting and infected body of the British-oriental opium trade (44–45).[11] Harold, like other culturally hybrid characters of the 1860s, embodies this threat—the orientalized British gentleman. Alicia Carroll points out the problematic imperial politics of the novel in Eliot's presentation of the orientalized Englishman who is both a Giaour and "an Oriental, you know" (237). Carroll argues that Harold's purchase of an enslaved Greek wife not only "participates in the . . . desecration of Greek culture which so infuriated Byron" but also reminds Victorians of the sensational 1851 Crystal Palace Exhibition of the painting by Hiram Powers entitled *The Greek Slave,* wherein a white Greek woman is exposed and sold to dark-skinned Turkish men (245). Ultimately, Carroll believes Eliot aligns him with—and thus critiques—Disraelian imperialism. As Carroll's reading suggests, Eliot's connection of his orientalized attributes to his very middle-class, very English father Jermyn problematizes a simple story of Easternized man invading the West. Still, Carroll argues that Turkey, especially in 1832, was seen as the very type of oppression.

Certainly, this is largely true. However, we must also remind ourselves of British complicity in Turkish oppression of the Greeks, British attempts to help Turkey consolidate their military, and British hatred of Turkey's enemy, Russia, all of which had contributed to complicate British attitudes toward Turkey by the 1860s—when *Felix Holt* was actually written. The British were also aware of the liberal, modernizing movement of many younger Turkish intellectuals. Turkey, like China, thus becomes a complex symbol of oriental despotism but also of British complicity and romantic nationalism. Eliot brings home oriental despotism to reside in the respectable English male, ruling through judicious medication of the population. Harold is the oriental drug dealer who would seduce and orientalize Esther, imprisoning her in his "rose satin" drawing room. Finally, Eliot links his oriental despotism explicitly to his denigration of the moral influence of and respect for women—Eliot commits her one historical misrepresentation in giving Harold a Greek slave as late as the 1830s, probably to make precisely that point. The British merchant who, with the Turks, dominates the Hellenic cradle of Western democracy, spuriously packages himself as a radical advocate of democracy in Britain.

And in Harold Transome, monstrously respectable, the quintessential

11. Cannon Schmitt, in *Alien Nation,* remarks that the English constructed themselves against the oriental specifically in light of their relationship to opium.

English gentleman "Giaour" and self-proclaimed "Oriental" whose son is born of a slave woman who was purchased, apparently for the purpose, we have indeed a Malthusian vision of "appropriately" moderated desire: "I never want anything I can't get," he says cheerfully. "Fond of sensual pleasures, but disinclined to all vice, and attached as a healthy, clearsighted person, to all conventional morality," Harold is not immune from desire but balanced by competing desires: "He was addicted at once to rebellion and conformity" (110). Clearly the temperate desire that dominated models of social engineering is not, for Eliot, enough alone to guarantee moral fitness.

Although many critics have read Harold as an orientalizing narrative, no one seems to have noticed the other oriental male in the novel. Dominic, Harold's servant, is, as Harold says, "of no country in particular. I don't know whether he is most of a Jew, a Greek, an Italian or a Spaniard," but "he's an affectionate fellow—I can trust to his attachment. That's a sort of human specimen that doesn't grow here in England" (37). In fact, he is wrong; his mother's English servant, Eliot's nostalgic representation of a holdover from more feudal days, has exactly that kind of devotion. But Dominic, whatever he is besides a splendid cook, is loyal and affectionate, and he plays the role of mother to Harry. This representation, of course, plays on another orientalist narrative—the effeminate male.[12] But if it reinforces stereotypes of Mediterranean passion and Northern rationality, it also tends to place tyranny on the side of cool calculation. Harold's monstrosity is not that he has the immoderate desires associated with orientalism but precisely that his desires can be satisfied—that they drive him on to no higher level of development, emotional or moral. That satisfaction becomes an end in itself in the same way that the desires created by capitalism and by addiction become ends in themselves.

The point for Eliot, as for Bentham, is to acknowledge desire and use it, harness it to social ends. These ends, however, are not mere material wealth or political power (as Felix says of the vote, "Not yet! Something else before all that"), but an Arnoldian vision of culture that transmutes mere appetite into an evolutionary force in the service of humanity. This vision of appetite and addiction brings together rich and poor as subject to the same misuse of appetite: of paupers, Felix explains in his "address to the working men" that they have "the worst vices of the worst rich—who are gamblers, sots, libertines," and "they are the multiplying brood begotten by parents who have been left without all teaching save that of a too craving body, without all well-being save the fading delusions of drugged beer and gin" (492). Eliot recommends culture as the substitute for drugs, urging her audience to foster and preserve "the treasure of refined needs" (495).

12. See Sara Suleri, for example.

Eliot rewrites the earlier social problem novel of the Chartist era, updating it to deal with the social and cultural concerns of the second Reform Bill period and giving it the conservative turn to culture (instead of domesticity) over politics that it would hardly have born earlier. She does so by combining the themes and characteristic scenes of the social problem novel (the riot, a courtroom scene reminiscent of *Mary Barton,* the election) with the plot elements of the sensation novel (the transgressive aristocratic woman with a secret, the blackmailer, the birth mystery plot, the misplaced inheritance). The metaphor of addiction becomes the glue to hold these disparate elements together, placing contemporary concerns about opium addiction, oriental corruption, and the transgressive working-class male and middle-class woman in a single unified narrative of desire gone wrong. However, Eliot also emphasizes the complexities of this desire—the desire that destroys the social fabric is the same desire that holds it together. Therefore, desire must neither be avoided nor overindulged nor even simply managed; it must be managed ethically, with a vision behind its direction beyond the immediate needs of the moment. Harold, unlike his mother, represents not simply the short-term gratification of desires but even what a socially blameless self-control leads to without a long-term vision of how one's personal desires fit into a larger sense of social responsibility.

Eliot also rewrites both the sensation novel, constructed by critics as a dangerous drug, and the social problem novel, which traditionally delineates the conditions that create unmanageable cravings, as a novel of psychological realism that ambivalently emphasizes a vision of common humanity over class and racial difference. Although Esther's melodramatic birth mystery plot resolves itself in favor of essentialized class differences—she always felt she was born with upper-class tastes, and voilà! she is, by birth, upper class—she resigns her class position and works among the poor with lower-middle-class Felix, whose origins are unabashedly working class. The aristocratic Harold, with his princely Eastern demeanor, is the son of the middle-class Jermyn—and shows it. The orientalized despot is not the sybarite who gluts his appetites but one who does not think beyond his appropriate level of comfort, even when that comfort is defined in socially approved terms. "Addiction" therefore comes to mean not only transgressive desire but also the trap of a too-complacent conformity.

Thus the aims of social problem novels that aspire toward economic or political solutions are linked with the transgressions that sensation novels breathlessly detail and denounce—both highlight what Eliot considers the problematic of desire. While political economists strive for a channeling of desire based on self-interest and sensation novels chart the wayward courses of desire gone wrong, both, for Eliot wrongly, focus on a social management of desire as an individualistic motive, whereas for Eliot, proper enculturation links individual desire to communitarian altruism. For Eliot, the "appropriately" desiring British gentleman who trusts the profit motive and a "healthy, active selfishness" is the dangerous despot, orientalized not by residence in Turkey but by his own disregard for anything larger than his own personal goals. Eliot's vision is thus essentially conservative. In her model of addiction, we can see the prehistory of today's readings of addiction as rooted in social problems. Finally, however, despite Eliot's careful social analysis of the contexts for drug abuse and addiction, she has no social solution to offer, defaulting to a familiar liberal prescription of individual self-discipline. (Perhaps unsurprisingly, this is still largely the solution offered today.)

In the addictive body, we see the threat to citizenship of a subject who has learned too well to desire but failed to benefit from the social by learning the techniques necessary to displace and contain that desire. But Eliot points to a critique not offered by Dickens's grotesque representations of desire out of control—she, like Arnold, hints that even the apparently good citizen can undermine the liberal ideal of cultural uplift, if that compliant citizen settles for an existence as a self-medicating philistine. The problems of desire are inherent to its nature, just as the body is inherently vulnerable. Liberalism itself is founded on a perpetual negotiation between desire and discipline, between the individual and the nation, between agency and socialization. That is both its weakness and its strength.

AFTERWORD

LIBERALISM AND ITS DISCONTENTS

> The same bare life that in the *ancien regime* was politically neutral and belonged to God . . . fully enters into the structure of the state and even becomes the earthly foundation of the state's legitimacy and sovereignty.
>
> —Giorgio Agamben, *Homo Sacer*

The articulation of fitness as a primary criterion for the franchise in the 1830s through the 1860s, even though fitness at this point still included a rental qualification, paved the way for a right to health. Fitness designated the child as a special category. Since the child could not choose where he lived or if he were educated, the development of fitness was not within his control. Education must be provided so the child could develop the basic literacy necessary to understand political issues; of course, education was also an opportunity for indoctrination into the elite view of political economy.[1] School alone, however, did not affect the child's living conditions.[2] If the ability to labor and thus gain the income status required for qualification was injured, obviously the child could not develop fitness and might also became an economic burden on the rate-paying citizenry. But additionally, if the child's health, which was viewed as prerequisite for the development of a minimal moral competence, depended on living conditions, then the living conditions necessary for the possibility of fitness must be provided for the developing citizen. As remains true today, the child became the site of a debate around entitlements and also a node of state interest in the realm of domestic privacy.

But (also as remains true today), liberalism infantilized every person or culture who did not fit into its view of the good citizen. By positing a universal "natural" subject, liberalism demanded that everyone who did not

1. See Marshall and Bottomore on this point.
2. For a discussion of education as a social right, see Bernard Harris.

fit the definition of this subject be seen as unnatural, deviant—or at least incompletely developed, a moral child. Darwin posited that all humans came from a single ancestor and that European civilization represented a high level of moral development that was itself predicated on the natural evolution of "social instincts." By a similar logic, non-European civilizations—and Europeans who did not fit into their own civilizations' notion of the "good citizen"—were seen as failures in natural development who had to be either coaxed back onto a proper developmental path or ruled with the paternal despotism appropriate to their infantile level of evolution.

The irony of this assumption is that it presupposes that the "individual" so prized under a liberal rule will be marked only by very minor and superficial differences: I like coffee, you like tea. Identity markers that may be constitutive of subjectivity—gender, class, race, religion—are still relegated to the private, although critiques of this division have been persistently mounted. Politics, in such a logic, becomes a rather narcissistic conversation about minor differences, the *real* business of state being so obviously agreed upon as to merit little discussion or even consciousness. Meanwhile, within the problematic of gender in liberal societies, residual structures of the public and private and the masculinity of the universal subject continue to plague women's attempts to gain political power. Rights feminists have often made their advances at the cost of suppressing women's difference from the universal subject, resulting, for example, in better access to labor opportunity at the expense of access to maternity and daycare benefits. On the other hand, the attempt to advance "women" as a category, often in response to the inadequacies of the aforementioned rights feminism, has often resulted in the suppression of racial, class, sexual, and ethnic differences. And the perpetuation of the public-private divide has meant that gains in one area have very often resulted in costs in another.[3] The split we have inherited between public and private, political and social, is not sustainable, but within liberalism there has not yet been a successful retheorization of the problem.[4]

Capitalism, it has been argued, (re)created the social sphere after the demise of feudalism, founding the very conditions of citizenship. Conversely, it has been argued that capitalism "just grew," and the conditions necessary

3. In the United States, for example, workfare programs designed to foster "independence" and possessive individualism are often poorly coordinated with childcare, resulting in excessive costs to mothers receiving "benefits," or marriage-advocacy policies that attempt to shore up the family result in increased exploitation of and violence against women within the home.

4. Once again, I am referring here to Western liberal states. As Partha Chatterjee has noted, the development of ideas of nation and of the private have progressed very differently in some other locations. For a discussion of those differences in Bengal, see Chatterjee, especially 72–75.

to this brilliant weed required economic freedoms of the constituents of the labor force and hence social freedoms mirroring them that gave birth to liberal conceptions of rights. Either way, liberal citizenship encodes the most basic tension within capitalism, its promise of exclusivity universally available. If capitalism motivated the creation of modern citizenship, its desiderata seem plainly in opposition to foundational citizens' rights now. Why neoconservatism and the dismantling of the welfare state? Why privatization of social services? Capitalism constructed the (first-world) citizen against its other, the pauper, and the English/British nation against its other, the colonies. But the empire has struck back.

In part, the first world has achieved its historically unstable prosperity, enabling mass consumption, by "outsourcing" poverty. Global late capitalism now struggles with its own necessary other, the "developing" world; the model of citizenship shows the fissures of its formation against the pressures of the new "massed" economic outcaste, as high-consuming nations are forced to confront their labor "slums" in Southeast Asia, Africa, Latin America, and so on. Whether (one) history "ends" as liberalism and capitalism saturate the globe, precipitating a necessary reconfiguration of relations of production, or whether liberal capitalist omnivorousness finds its final check in confrontation with indigestible Othernesses, it seems clear that many of the assumptions underlying today's Victorian forms of liberalism will not bear the strain of current developments. It remains to be seen what a political philosophy that would revise some of these foundational fictions while retaining other, perhaps still viable, values would look like, what vision of the body and self, and what art, it will produce.

Among theorists who have attempted this task, Richard Rorty provides an important example of the difficulties these thinkers face. His utopian postmodern liberalism seems a step away from traditional individualism, advocating a decentered subject who understands his or her position as constructed. He argues that such a subject would have an ironic relationship with his or her "self," understanding it as provisional and situational, liable to change with circumstance. This subject would easily shed its more private subject positions when called to debate public and political matters. Indeed, however, such ironic distance seems rather exclusively the purview of elites.[5] Light irony, as George Eliot remarked, is an expensive production. It is rare

5. And, I should add, first-world elites, though I also want to clarify that my own discussion claims relevance only to late modernity in the United Kingdom and the United States. Even in other Western democratic societies, these debates have developed quite differently, and in other societies the strategic usefulness of liberal discourse may make for very different investments in different historical moments. It is telling that Rorty reads only white European men in *Contingency, Irony, and Solidarity*.

that the subaltern can afford to be—if, indeed, he or she would want or be able to be—other than in earnest in defending his or her commitments. And sometimes the subaltern may be, of necessity, closer to the kind of radically situated self that critic of liberalism Michael Sandel describes than first-world elites. The radically situated self is entrenched in a single subject position related largely to membership in one community and defines priorities more by communitarian commitments than by notions of the individual; such a self often does not move between multiple subject positions without paying a high price. That situatedness may be a condition of economic and cultural subalternity, as well as a deliberate choice (Native Americans attempting to preserve traditional communities on reservations come to mind).[6] It is precisely what they might perceive as a value-neutral sense of irony and contingency that such subjects are rejecting.

Rorty, of course, does restrict this ironic stance to the intelligentsia in his ideal state, and strictly to civil society rather than politics; "irony" he notes, "seems inherently a private matter." His "masses" would be "commonsensically nominalist and historicist" (87). But it is neither the "intelligentsia" nor the majority in the United States or United Kingdom who poses the most obvious problem for global liberalism, but the subaltern, at home and abroad. Rorty is persuasive when he bases his liberalism on the avoidance of cruelty within a recognition that all circumstances, including those defining cruelty, are contingent. But finally, we are faced with the question of what happens when powerful societies or groups "redefine" less powerful ones, and Rorty can offer only the old solutions: "we need to distinguish between redescription for public and private purposes" (91) in order to avoid "humiliating" less powerful others, who are again described as immature: "Consider what happens when a child's precious possessions . . . are redescribed as 'trash' and thrown away. Or . . . are made to look ridiculous alongside the possessions of another, richer, child. Something like that presumably happens to a primitive culture when it is conquered by a more advanced one" (89–90).

My point here is not to denigrate Rorty's careful and often compelling argument by focusing on an unfortunate choice of metaphor but to point out that this metaphor is deeply embedded in the history of liberalism's conceptions of the Other. The Other is assumed to use a universal standard of evaluation that dictates the intuitive judgment that first-world, mainstream

6. I am aware of the difficulties associated with the adoption of a binary of oppressor/oppressed, liberal subject/other. However, although these are not essential but situational characteristics, in any given encounter of the type defined above a power difference can be defined, at least within the boundaries of the particular situation, usefully in those terms. It behooves us, as we attempt to attend to the complexities of such encounters, to recall this basic disparity.

"toys"—customs, goods, and values—are better. This is the root of the difficulty that liberalism faces when it encounters the Other; because we *are* liberals, we have to care about another's power to define her or himself, yet the whole edifice of the liberal state depends on a certain homogeneity in the conception of the self that is profoundly challenged by unassimilable difference, not to mention subalternity. Although liberal universalism defines itself against an "outside," it also posits that all that difference is ultimately assimilable, as inessential to the deep structure of the self. We do not, under current global economic conditions, have the option to (nor is anyone choosing to), as L. T. Hobhouse suggested in his landmark statement *Liberalism* in 1911, simply leave the Other alone.[7] Infantilizing the Other is the move that enables liberal "Western" states to ignore the incoherence of our position—a politically effective move in the short term, perhaps, but not, finally, a democratic or even a liberal one per se.

The major challenge to liberal universalism within the United States and the United Kingdom is, of course, the increasing cultural heterogeneity of the population and the claims of resultant counterpublics.[8] Scholars who have attempted to address these changes argue that a shifting, situationally specific and avowedly imaginary boundary constituted with a language of (socially constituted) rights versus responsibilities rather than public and private per se could provide a valuable way to continue a form of liberal society in which we are constituted as subjects and which we therefore appropriately value highly. Movement away from a grand theory of liberalism toward a looser set of constantly negotiated values that can operate as a rough guide in a case-by-case approach to political situations—what Gayatri Chakravorty Spivak calls strategies, rather than theories—may be the only way we can approach the challenges of dealing with difference.

This move leads us again in the direction of Rorty, or of Chantal Mouffe (and Ernesto Laclau), who have decoupled the concept of the public sphere of liberal, reasoned discourse from its link with capitalism. However, as Rorty and Mouffe imply, we must eliminate the assumption of liberal universality and recognize that there are situations and cultures in which liberal assumptions are not useful; that there are other valuable and viable ways to organize

7. This text was foundational in articulating the "New Liberalism"—a term coined to describe the work of political thinkers such as L. T. Hobhouse and T. H. Green in the early twentieth century, who embraced philosophical liberalism while rejecting classical economic liberalism and sought balance between the rights of the individual and the claims of communities.

8. See, for example, John Gray (305 and passim). He argues that this has resulted in the demise of liberalism as a theoretically viable construct, but that what remains is the viable legacy of civil society.

both states and human experience (see Gray 314–28, Mouffe 145–52). This does not mean that individual liberal states must slide into relativism; as Mouffe argues, it does mean taking seriously the fact that neither the state nor liberal values can be neutral and that arbitrating between groups is both difficult and value charged—and therefore thoroughly political. It does mean giving up a Habermasian Enlightenment epistemology (though even Mouffe and Rorty seem in practice to privilege reason and debate as a near-absolute value). And thus it does mean, once again, that liberal debate will finally fail to be an adequate response for many cultural encounters. As early as 1911 Hobhouse argued that "to destroy tribal custom by introducing conceptions of individual property, the free disposal of land and the free purchase of gin may be the handiest method for the expropriator. . . . If men say equality, they mean oppression by forms of justice. If they say tutelage, they appear to mean the kind of tutelage extended to the fattened goose" (20). In nearly a century, we have improved little on Hobhouse's articulation of the problem.

There are those theorists who would prefer to dispense with the state or even a global government entirely, such as Giorgio Agamben. Agamben agrees with Foucault that modernity has seen the full instantiation of biopolitics. Biopolitics, he believes, reached its logical extreme in Nazi concentration camps, wherein, as Arendt says, the penetration of privacy and the body by state power is absolute. He argues, however, that the seeds of this tendency existed at the very inception of Western political thought, in which the denial of the *oikos* or the domestic and of *zoe,* or what he terms "bare life," within the sphere of politics paradoxically made bare life and power over it the unacknowledged basis of all forms of sovereignty and citizenship. He claims that "only a politics that will have learned to take the fundamental biopolitical fracture of the West into account" will be able to stem the "thanotic" tendencies of biopolitics to absolute domination and destruction (*Homo Sacer* 181). Such a politics, he envisions, would ultimately enable people to dispense with a state altogether in favor of a community in which persons would not need to be conceived within any "representable condition of belonging" (*Coming Community* 86). Such a community would be founded on a human condition in which there was no division between the political and bare life, and no sovereignty as we now understand it.

I have said that the assumption of a universal subject and the splitting of public and private mystify the nature of the state and its tutelary role and, by rendering the subject it constructs "natural," place (or attempt to place) this subject beyond critique and revision and homogenize the political, public sphere of debate in such a way as to deny access to Others, in whatever way constituted. However, in objecting to the mystification of the state's tutelary role, and in critiquing some of the values that it has historically inculcated, I do not object to the tutelary role of the state itself. All states—fascist, Marxist, democratic—perform such a role, whether through the exercise of naked power or the mobilization of consent. To assume that they should not, that human beings should develop in absolute freedom from state or even social tutelage, requires precisely the assumption that there is a preexisting self that society deforms.

I make this fairly obvious point because, in critics' zeal to uncover the mechanisms by which power often shapes the subject, an evaluation of the effects and aims of such power is sometimes lacking. Surveillance is not all equally bad, just as "resistance" is not all equally subversive and "subversion" is itself not uniformly valuable. The state and political sphere may be a proper place for certain principles to be valorized, where they can be debated openly and where appeal to the rule of law is possible for groups that perceive themselves to be affected negatively. Perhaps better that the state should be the site of such debate than so-called civil society, whose exercise of real institutional power is often masked by the public/private divide so that no appeal for protection is possible—such were the problems, for example, that led U.S. lawmakers to pass laws in protection of minorities' rights against employment discrimination rights that are continually endangered at the levels of both practice and legislation. On the other hand, though I am sympathetic to Michael Walzer's arguments about the recurring need for communitarian critique in liberalism, I am also skeptical of some localist communitarian stances. To suppose that local communities are inherently more valuable than a community defined by the state is based on assumptions that are not entirely clear to me; after all, a culture that shapes its discussion of values at the state level—with a due regard for dissent within subgroups and protection of their access to the public sphere—does not necessarily have to be a less worthy site of community identity than a region, religion, or ethnicity.[9]

9. Partha Chatterjee has advanced a reading of Indian nationalism as proceeding through a different narrative. The colonial state destroyed the "fuzziness" and multiplicity of existing community affiliations in order to fix colonial subjects within certain "community" identities that were understood as—and structurally compelled to be—fixed and exclusive, to be ordered and subsumed within the state. Indian nationalism at certain points, he argues, opposed this new sense of community: Gandhi, for example, used a rhetoric that was "antimodernist, antiindividualist, even anticapitalist. The attempt is . . . to find, against the grand narrative of history itself, the cultural resources through which people, living in different, contextually defined, communities, can coexist . . . within larger political units." In other words, the rhetoric of nation was used against the homogenizing tendency displayed by the rhetoric of the liberal nation-state in Europe. However, "this other narrative is again violently interrupted once the postcolonial nation state attempts to resume its journey along the

As strategies for resistance against harmful hegemonic forces, localism may be extremely useful, but sometimes the most passionate local investments can be the site of very ugly modes of identification based on violence and exclusion. Further, these same modes may be collaborative with those same hegemonic forces they appear to resist.[10] If reports of the death of history have been greatly exaggerated, so has the postmortem of liberalism perhaps been hasty.

I also have (unsurprisingly) no proposal for a remedy to the difficulty I have identified—a problematic that has both enabled liberal advances and limited their efficacy. As I have already indicated, I believe we are not yet ready to move beyond the state, and I find the romanticism in some of Giorgio Agamben's formulations troubling: his idealization of pure presence, of an unmediated subjectivity in a millennial "coming community." One serious problem with his conception is that, much like liberal universalism, it assumes that local identities, or "representable conditions of belonging," should be irrelevant in the ideal community. But Agamben's effort to create the conditions of possibility to at least think such a community—or to think beyond what we have—demands our careful attention. And perhaps the very fact that he leads us back to a universalism-through-the-back-door indicates that we should rethink the usefulness of liberal values. Amanda Anderson, in *The Way We Argue Now,* has called for a return not only to a carefully theorized and pragmatic liberal cosmopolitanism but also, more controversially, to an openly avowed embrace of its normative and evaluative elements. After all, most of the challenges to liberalism in the West have relied implicitly or explicitly on norms of justice developed out of liberalism itself; to the extent that this is true, the question then becomes one of government structure and political practice rather than goals or values. Anderson aligns herself, with some reservations, with positions argued by Habermasians such as Seyla Benhabib—toward a liberal discourse ethics informed by a contingent universalism. However, Anderson focuses her attention solely on the political opposition between local (largely ethnic) identities and universal ones rather than on the question of public and private per se; she elides the important

---

trajectory of world historical development. The modern state, embedded as it is within the universal narrative of capital, cannot recognize within its jurisdiction any form of community except the single, determinate, demographically enumerable form of the nation" (238). In this way, he argues, the parochial history of Europe has and continues, through the legacies of colonialism, to replicate itself in countries and communities where quite different practices and concepts might otherwise have emerged. When I use the term "communitarian" above, I am speaking of some specific groups in specific historical circumstances, rather than using it in this larger theoretical sense within which, as Chatterjee argues, the possibilities have not been fully explored.

10. Some of the heinous practices enacted under supposedly liberal governments, such as sterilization of the genetically "undesirable" in the United States and the United Kingdom, have been justified with communitarian arguments. See Desmond King for an extended discussion.

question of how one comes to the conversation in the first place.[11] One might say, however, that if liberalism has tended to suppress such identities unless or until they can become sites of political identification and mobilization, it has also, finally, provided a mechanism for those sites to be recognized beyond that point in time. As do many critics, I believe that within the utopian elements of liberal Enlightenment thought is something valuable, as well as dangerous.

Agamben points to the possibility of a modest beginning. In order to foster the "emergence of a field of research beyond the terrain defined by the intersection of politics and philosophy, medico-biological sciences and jurisprudence," he offers a Foucauldian solution: we must first "examine how it was possible for something like a bare life to be conceived within these disciplines" and trace the historical development of our current situation (*Homo Sacer* 188). However, as bare life is endemic to any conception of sovereignty for Agamben, he wishes to move beyond sovereignty itself. I would argue that as the creation of bare life is endemic to sovereignty, the ability to critique and resist this category must already have come as well from within the structure in which it is conceived. To transcend our episteme, it is necessary first to understand how it formed and functions; it is also necessary to evaluate what within it has continued to be of value. This volume offers a step toward this project of historical analysis.

11. Anderson's otherwise admirable book has a persistent tendency to elide the status of justice within the debate she critiques, conflating it with questions of affect.

WORKS CITED

Note: In the parenthetical citations, *Hansard's* indicates *Hansard's Parliamentary Debates.*

Acton, Lord. "Nationality." Reprinted in *Mapping the Nation,* ed. Gopal Balakrishnan. New York: Verso, 1996. 17–38.

Agamben, Giorgio. *Homo Sacer: Sovereign Power and Bare Life.* Trans. Daniel Heller-Roazen. Stanford, CA: Stanford University Press, 1998.

———. *The Coming Community.* Trans. Michael Hardt. Minneapolis: University of Minnesota Press, 1993.

Alborn, Timothy L. "A Plague Upon Your Health: Commercial Crisis and Epidemic Disease in Victorian England." *Biology as Society, Society as Biology: Metaphors,* ed. Sabine Maasen, Peter Weingart, and Everett Mendelssohn. Dordrecht, Netherlands: Kluwer Academic Press, 1995. 281–310.

Anderson, Amanda. *The Powers of Distance: Cosmopolitanism and the Cultivation of Detachment.* Princeton, NJ: Princeton University Press, 2001.

Anderson, Benedict. *Imagined Communities.* 1983. Rev. ed. London: Verso, 1991.

Arendt, Hannah. *The Human Condition.* Chicago: University of Chicago Press, 1958.

Armstrong, Nancy. *Desire and Domestic Fiction: A Political History of the Novel.* Oxford: Oxford University Press, 1987.

Barrett Browning, Elizabeth. *Aurora Leigh.* Chicago: Academy Chicago Publishers, 1979.

Beiner, Ronald. *What's the Matter with Liberalism?* Berkeley: University of California Press, 1992.

Bellamy, Richard. "Pluralism, Liberal Constitutionalism and Democracy: A Critique of John Rawls's (Meta) Political Liberalism." In *The Liberal Political Tradition: Contemporary Reappraisals,* ed. James Meadowcroft. Cheltenham, UK: Edward Elgar Press. 77–100.

Bentham, Jeremy. *The Principles of Morals and Legislation.* Buffalo, NY: Prometheus Books, 1988.

Bhabha, Homi K. "DissemiNation: Time, Narrative, and the Margins of the Modern Nation." In *Nation and Narration,* ed. Homi K. Bhabha. London: Routledge, 1990. 298–300.

Biagini, Eugenio F., ed. *Citizenship and Community: Liberals, Radicals, and Collective*

Identities in the British Isles, 1865–1931. New York: Cambridge University Press, 1996.

Bourdieu, Pierre. *Distinction: A Social Judgment of the Critique of Taste.* Trans. Richard Nice. Cambridge, MA: Harvard University Press, 1984.

———. *Outline of a Theory of Practice.* Trans. Richard Nice. Cambridge, MA: Harvard University Press, 1977.

Boyd, Nancy. *Three Victorian Women Who Changed Their World: Josephine Butler, Octavia Hill, Florence Nightingale.* Oxford: Oxford University Press, 1982.

Braddon, Mary Elizabeth. *Lady Audley's Secret.* Oxford: Oxford University Press, 1991.

Brantlinger, Patrick. *The Spirit of Reform: British Literature and Politics, 1832–1867.* Cambridge, MA: Harvard University Press, 1977.

———. *Fictions of State: Culture and Credit in Britain, 1694–1994.* Ithaca, NY: Cornell University Press, 1996.

Bushnan, J. Stevenson. *Cholera and Its Cures: An Historical Sketch.* London: Wm. S. Orr and Co., 1850.

Carroll, Alicia. "The Giaour's Campaign: Desire and the Other in Felix Holt, the Radical." *Novel* 30.2 (Winter 1997): 237–58.

Chadwick, Edwin. 1842. *Report on the Labouring Population of Great Britain.* Edited with an introduction by M. W. Flinn. Edinburgh: Edinburgh University Press, 1965.

Chadwick, Edwin, and Southwood Smith. "Report." Irish University Press Parliamentary Papers 1849, *Cholera* I. August 14, 1850.

Chase, Karen, and Michael Levenson. *The Spectacle of Intimacy: A Public Life for the Victorian Family.* Princeton, NJ: Princeton University Press.

Chatterjee, Partha. *The Nation and Its Fragments: Colonial and Postcolonial Histories.* Princeton, NJ: Princeton University Press, 1993.

Colley, Linda. *Britons: Forging the Nation, 1707–1837.* New Haven, CT: Yale University Press, 1992.

Collins, Wilkie. *The Woman in White.* Peterborough, ON: Broadview Press, 1999.

Daunton, M. J. *House and Home in the Victorian City: Working-Class Housing, 1850–1914.* London: Edward Arnold, 1983.

David, Deirdre. *Fictions of Resolution in Three Victorian Novels.* New York: Columbia University Press, 1981.

Delaporte, François. *Disease and Civilization: The Cholera in Paris, 1832.* Trans. Arthur Goldhammer; foreword by Paul Rabinow. Cambridge, MA: MIT Press, 1986.

Deleuze, Gilles. Foreword to Jacques Donzelot, *The Policing of Families.* Trans. Robert Hurley. New York: Pantheon, 1979.

Dellamora, Richard. *Friendship's Bonds: Democracy and the Novel in Victorian England.* Philadelphia: University of Pennsylvania Press, 2004.

Dickens, Charles. *Bleak House.* 1853. Oxford: Oxford University Press, 1996.

———. *The Mystery of Edwin Drood.* 1870. Oxford: Oxford University Press, 1956.

———. *Our Mutual Friend.* 1865. Oxford: Oxford University Press, 1952.

Dimock, Wai Chee. "Class, Gender and a History of Metonymy." In *Rethinking Class: Literary Studies and Social Formations,* ed. Wai Chee Dimock and Michael T. Gilmore. New York: Columbia University Press, 1994. 57–104.

Dimock, Wai Chee, and Michael T. Gilmore. "Introduction." In *Rethinking Class: Literary Studies and Social Formations,* ed. Wai Chee Dimock and Michael T. Gilmore.

New York: Columbia University Press, 1994. 1–14.
"Discussion of Professor Kerr's Paper." *RIBA Journal of Proceedings* (1866–67): 48–81.
Disraeli, Benjamin. *Coningsby.* 1844. London: Dent, 1963.
———. *Sybil, or, The Two Nations.* 1845. London and New York: John Lane, The Bodley Head, 1905.
Donzelot, Jacques. *The Policing of Families.* Trans. Robert Hurley. New York: Pantheon, 1979.
Durey, Michael. *The Return of the Plague: British Society and the Cholera, 1831–2.* Dublin: Gill and Macmillan Humanities Press, 1979.
Elias, Norbert. *The Civilizing Process: The Development of Manners. Changes in the Code of Conduct and Feeling in Early Modern Times.* Trans. Edmund Jephcott. New York: Urizen Books, 1978.
Eliot, George. *Felix Holt, the Radical.* 1866. New York: Penguin, 1995.
———. *The Mill on the Floss.* 1860. Oxford: Oxford University Press, 1998.
Elliot, Dorice Williams. *The Angel Out of the House: Philanthropy and Gender in Nineteenth-Century England.* Charlottesville: University Press of Virginia, 2002.
Evans, Richard. "Epidemics and Revolutions: Cholera in Nineteenth Century-Europe." *Past and Present* 120 (1988): 123–46.
Farr, William. "Influence of Elevation on Fatality of Cholera." *Journal of the Royal Statistical Society* 15 (1852): 155–83.
———. *Report on the Mortality of Cholera in England, 1848–49.* London, 1852.
———. *Vital Statistics. A Memorial Volume of Selections from the Reports and Writings of William Farr. With an Introduction by Mervyn Susser and Abraham Adelstein.* Metuchen, NJ: Scarecrow Press, 1975.
Finn, Margot C. *After Chartism: Class and Nation in English Radical Politics, 1848–1874.* Cambridge: Cambridge University Press, 1993.
Flint, Kate. *The Woman Reader, 1837–1914.* Oxford: Oxford University Press.
Foucault, Michel. "Governmentality." In *The Foucault Effect: Studies in Governmentality,* ed. Graham Burchell, Colin Gordon, and Peter Miller. Chicago: University of Chicago Press, 1991. 87–104.
Fraser, Nancy. "Rethinking the Public Sphere: A Contribution to the Critique of Actually Existing Democracy." *Social Text* 8–9 (1990): 56–80.
Frazer, Elizabeth. "Feminism and Liberalism." In *The Liberal Political Tradition: Contemporary Reappraisals,* ed. James Meadowcroft. Cheltenham, UK: Edward Elgar Press. 138–58.
Gallagher, Catherine. "The Bioeconomics of *Our Mutual Friend.*" In *Subject to History,* ed. David Simpson. Ithaca, NY: Cornell University Press, 1991. 47–69.
Gaskell, Elizabeth. *Mary Barton.* 1848. Oxford: Oxford University Press, 1998.
———. *North and South.* 1855. New York: Penguin, 1995.
Giddens, Anthony. *The Constitution of Society: Outline of the Theory of Structuration.* Los Angeles: University of California Press, 1984.
Gilbert, Pamela K. *Disease, Desire and the Body in Victorian Women's Popular Novels.* Cambridge: Cambridge University Press, 1997.
———. *Mapping the Victorian Social Body.* Albany: SUNY Press, 2004.
———. "'A Sinful and Suffering Nation': Cholera and the Evolution of Medical and Religious Authority in Britain, 1832–1866." *Nineteenth-Century Prose* 25.1 (Spring 1998): 35–59.

Godwin, George. *London Shadows: A Glance at the Homes of the Thousands.* 1854. London: George Routledge and Co.

———. *Town Swamps and Social Bridges. The Sequel to* A Glance at the Homes of the Thousands. London: Routledge, Warnes and Routledge, 1859.

Goodlad, Lauren. *Victorian Literature and the Victorian State.* Baltimore: Johns Hopkins University Press, 2003.

Gottfried, Paul Edward. *After Liberalism: Mass Democracy in the Managerial State.* Princeton, NJ: Princeton University Press, 1999.

Gotto, Edward. "Report on Church Lane and Carrier Street, St. Giles" (July 7, 1849). Public Records Office.

Gray, John. *Post-Liberalism: Studies in Political Thought.* New York: Routledge, 1993.

Gunn, J. A. W. "Public Interest." In *Political Innovation and Conceptual Change.* Cambridge: Cambridge University Press, 1989. 194–210.

Gurney, Michael S. "Disease as Device: The Role of Smallpox in *Bleak House.*" *Literature and Medicine* 9 (1990): 79–92.

Guy, Josephine. *The Victorian Social-Problem Novel: The Market, the Individual, and Communal Life.* New York: St. Martin's Press, 1996.

Habermas, Jürgen. *The Structural Transformation of the Public Sphere.* Trans. Thomas Burger, with Frederick Lawrence. Cambridge, MA: MIT Press, 1991.

Hall, Catherine, Keith McClelland, and Jane Rendall, eds. *Defining the Victorian Nation: Class, Gender and the British Reform Act of 1867.* Cambridge: Cambridge University Press, 2000.

Harding, Geoffrey. *Opiate Addiction, Morality and Medicine: From Moral Illness to Pathological Disease.* New York: St. Martin's Press, 1988.

Harris, Bernard. *The Origins of the British Welfare State: Social Welfare in England and Wales, 1800–1945.* Basingstoke: Palgrave, 2004.

Harrison, Mark. *Public Health in British India: Anglo-Indian Preventive Medicine, 1859–1914.* Cambridge: Cambridge University Press, 1994.

Hill, Octavia. 1875. *Homes of the London Poor, Octavia Hill and The Bitter Cry of Outcast London, Andrew Mearns.* London: Frank Cass and Co, Ltd., 1970.

———. *Our Common Land and Other Short Essays.* London: Macmillan, 1877.

Hobhouse, L. T. *Liberalism and Other Writings.* Ed. James Meadowcroft. Cambridge: Cambridge University Press, 1994.

Hoover, Terry Davis, et al. *A Guest in My Home.* Published through the collaborative efforts of the Family and Community Health, and Children and Families Program Office; the Ounce of Prevention Fund of Florida; and the Bureau of Student Services and Exceptional Education, Florida Department of Education, 1996.

Ignatieff, Michael. "The Myth of Citizenship." In *Theorizing Citizenship,* ed. Ronald Beiner. Albany: SUNY Press, 1995. 53–78.

Joyce, Patrick. *Democratic Subjects: The Self and the Social in Nineteenth-Century England.* Cambridge: Cambridge University Press, 1994.

———. *Visions of the People: Industrial England and the Question of Class, 1848–1914.* Cambridge: Cambridge University Press, 1991.

Kandall, Stephen R. *Substance and Shadow: Women and Addiction in the United States.* Cambridge, MA: Harvard University Press, 1996.

Kerr, Robert. "On the Problem of Providing Dwellings for the Poor in Towns." Lecture delivered before the Royal Institute of British Architects. *RIBA Journal of Proceedings*

(1866–67): 37–47.

King, Desmond S. *In the Name of Liberalism: Illiberal Social Policy in the United States and Britain.* Oxford: Oxford University Press, 1999.

Kingsley, Charles. *Alton Locke, Tailor and Poet: An Autobiography.* With a prefatory memoir by Thomas Hughes. New York: American Publishers Corp., [189-?].

Koven, Seth. "Borderlands: Women, Voluntary Action and Child Welfare in Britain, 1840–1914." *Mothers of a New World,* ed. Seth Koven and Sonya Michel. London: Routledge, 1993. 94–135.

———. *Slumming: Social and Sexual Politics in Victorian London.* Princeton, NJ: Princeton University Press, 2004.

Kucich, John. *Excess and Restraint in the Novels of Charles Dickens.* Athens: University of Georgia Press, 1981.

Ladies Sanitary Association. "The Use of Pure Water." 14th ed. London: Jarrold and Sons, [n.d., probably mid- to late 1860s].

Langland, Elizabeth. "Enclosure Acts: Framing Women's Bodies in Braddon's *Lady Audley's Secret.*" In *Beyond Sensation: Mary Elizabeth Braddon in Context,* ed. Marlene Tromp, Pamela Gilbert, and Aeron Haynie. New York: SUNY Press, 2000. 3–16.

———. *Nobody's Angels: Middle-Class Women and Domestic Ideology in Victorian Culture.* Ithaca, NY: Cornell University Press, 1995.

Leighninger, Leslie, and James Midgley. "United States of America." In *International Handbook on Social Work Theory and Practice,* ed. Nazneen S. Mayadas, Thomas D. Watts, and Doreen Elliott. Westport, CT: Greenwood Press, 1997. 9–28.

Lewis, Jane. "Presidential Address: Family Provision of Health and Welfare in the Mixed Economy of Care in the Late Nineteenth and Twentieth Centuries." *Social History of Medicine* 8.1 (April 1995): 1–16.

Malthus, Thomas Robert. *An Essay on the Principle of Population.* 1798. Oxford: Oxford University Press, 1999.

Marshall, T. H., and Tom Bottomore. *Citizenship and Social Class.* London: Pluto Press, 1992.

Marx, Karl. *The Class Struggles in France, 1848–1850.* Trans. Henry Kuhn. New York: New York Labor News, 1967.

———. *Marx-Engels: Selected Correspondence.* London: Martin Lawrence, 1936.

McClelland, Keith. "'England's Greatness, the Working Man.'" In *Defining the Victorian Nation: Class, Gender and the British Reform Act of 1867,* ed. Catherine Hall, Keith McClelland, and Jane Rendall. Cambridge: Cambridge University Press, 2000. 71–118.

McClintock, Anne. *Imperial Leather: Race, Gender, and Sexuality in the Colonial Contest.* New York: Routledge, 1995.

McCormack, Kathleen. *George Eliot and Intoxication: Dangerous Drugs for the Condition of England.* London: Macmillan, 2000.

———. "George Eliot and the Pharmakon: Dangerous Drugs for the Condition of England." *Victorians Institute Journal* 14 (1986): 35–52.

McKee, Patricia. *Public and Private: Gender, Class and the British Novel (1764–1878).* Minneapolis: University of Minnesota Press, 1997.

Mehta, Uday Singh. *Liberalism and Empire: A Study in Nineteenth-Century British Liberal Thought.* Chicago: University of Chicago Press, 1999.

Milligan, Barry. *Pleasures and Pains: Opium and the Orient in Nineteenth-Century British*

Culture. Charlottesville: University Press of Virginia, 1995.

Milton, Heather. "The Hand, the Head, and the Heart Meet Face to Face: Representations of Masculinity in *North and South.*" Unpublished paper, 1998.

Morris, Lydia. *Dangerous Classes: The Underclass and Social Citizenship.* London: Routledge, 1994.

Morris, R. J. *Cholera 1832: The Social Response to an Epidemic.* London: Croom Helm, 1976.

Mort, Frank. *Dangerous Sexualities: Medico-Moral Politics in England since 1830.* London: Routledge & Kegan Paul, 1987.

Mouffe, Chantal. *The Return of the Political.* New York: Verso, 1993.

O'Gorman, Frank. *Voters, Patrons, and Parties: The Unreformed Electoral System of Hanoverian England, 1734–1832.* Oxford: Oxford University Press, 1989.

Oldfield, Adrian. *Citizenship and Community: Civic Republicanism and the Modern World.* London: Routledge, 1990.

Oliphant, Margaret. *Miss Marjoribanks.* New York: Garland Publishers, 1976.

Parry, J. P. *The Rise and Fall of Liberal Government in Victorian Britain.* New Haven, CT: Yale University Press, 1993.

Parsinnen, Terry M. *Secret Passions, Secret Remedies: Narcotic Drugs in British Society, 1820–1930.* Philadelphia: Institute for the Study of Human Issues, 1883.

Pateman, Carole. *The Problem of Political Obligation: A Critical Analysis of Liberal Theory.* New York: Wiley, 1979.

Payne, Malcolm. "United Kingdom." In *International Handbook on Social Work Theory and Practice,* ed. Nazneen S. Mayadas, Thomas D. Watts, and Doreen Elliott Westport, CT: Greenwood Press, 1997. 161–83.

Pelling, Margaret. *Cholera, Fever and English Medicine, 1825–1865.* Oxford: Oxford University Press, 1978.

Pitkin, Hanna Fenichel. *The Attack of the Blob: Hannah Arendt's Concept of the Social.* Chicago: University of Chicago Press, 1998.

———. "Representation." In *Political Innovation and Conceptual Change.* Cambridge: Cambridge University Press, 1989. 132–54.

Plotz, John. *The Crowd: British Literature and Public Politics.* Berkeley: University of California Press, 2000.

Pocock, J. G. A. "The Ideal of Citizenship since Classical Times." In *Theorizing Citizenship,* ed. Ronald Beiner. Albany: SUNY Press, 1995. 29–52.

Poovey, Mary. *Making a Social Body: British Cultural Formation, 1830–1864.* Chicago: University of Chicago Press, 1995.

———. "The Social Constitution of Class: Toward a History of Classificatory Thinking." In *Rethinking Class: Literary Studies and Social Formations,* ed.,Wai Chee Dimock and Michael T. Gilmore. New York: Columbia University Press, 1994. 15–56.

Procacci, Giovanna. "Social Economy and the Government of Poverty." In *The Foucault Effect: Studies in Governmentality,* ed. Graham Burchell, Colin Gordon, and Peter Miller. Chicago: University of Chicago Press, 1991. 151–68.

Prochaska, Frank K. *Women and Philanthropy in Nineteenth-Century England.* Oxford: Clarendon Press, 1980.

"The Public Health Bill." *The Times* (July 28, 1866): 7–8.

Rawls, John. *A Theory of Justice.* Rev. ed. Cambridge, MA: Belknap Press of Harvard University Press, 1999.

Richards, Thomas. *The Imperial Archive: Knowledge and the Fantasy of Empire.* London: Verso, 1993.

Riley, Denise. *"Am I That Name?" Feminism and the Category of "Women" in History.* London: Macmillan, 1988.

Roberts, Henry, F.S.A. *The Dwellings of the Labouring Classes, their arrangement and construction, illustrated by a reference to the Model Houses of the Society for Improving the Condition of the Labouring Classes, and other buildings recently erected: being An Essay, read January 21, 1850, at the Royal Society of British Architects.* London: The Society for Improving the Condition of the Labouring Classes, 1850.

Roberts, Henry. *Home Reform.* London: Seeley's, Nisbet et al., 1855.

Robertson, David. *Class and the British Electorate.* Oxford: Basil Blackwell, 1984.

Rodger, Richard. *Housing in Urban Britain, 1780–1914: Class Capitalism and Construction.* London: Macmillan, 1989.

Rorty, Richard. *Contingency, Irony, and Solidarity.* Cambridge: Cambridge University Press, 1989.

Rose, Nikolas. *Powers of Freedom: Reframing Political Thought.* Cambridge: Cambridge University Press, 1999.

Rosenberg, Charles. *Explaining Epidemics and Other Studies in the History of Medicine.* Cambridge: Cambridge University Press, 1992.

Sandel, Michael. *Liberalism and the Limits of Justice.* Cambridge: Cambridge University Press, 1982.

Schmitt, Cannon. *Alien Nation: Nineteenth-Century Gothic Fictions and English Nationality.* Philadelphia: University of Pennsylvania Press, 1997.

Schwarzbach, F. S. "*Bleak House:* The Social Pathology of Urban Life." *Journal of Literature and Medicine* 9 (1990): 93–104.

SDUK (Society for the Diffusion of Useful Knowledge). *The Working Man's Companion. The Physician. 1. The Cholera.* London: Charles Knight, 1832.

Spivak, Gayatri Chakravorty. "Can the Subaltern Speak?" in Cary Nelson and Larry Grossberg, eds. *Marxism and the Interpretation of Culture.* Chicago: University of Illinois Press, 1988. 271–313.

Stallybrass, Peter, and Allon White. *The Politics and Poetics of Transgression.* Ithaca, NY: Cornell University Press, 1986.

Steig, Michael. "Dickens's Excremental Vision." *Victorian Studies* 8.3 (1970): 339–54.

Suleri, Sara. *The Rhetoric of English India.* Chicago: University of Chicago Press, 1992.

Sussman, Herbert L. *Victorian Masculinities: Manhood and Masculine Poetics in Early Victorian Literature and Art.* Cambridge: Cambridge University Press, 1995.

Sutherland, John, Esq. "General Board of Health. Report on the Sanitary Condition of the Epidemic Districts in the United Parishes of St. Giles and St. George, Bloomsbury, with special reference to the threatened visitation of epidemic cholera." London: George E. Eyre and William Spottiswoode, 1852.

Tarn, J. N. *Working-Class Housing in 19th-Century Britain.* London: Lund Humphries, 1971.

Thomas, David Wayne. *Cultivating Victorians: Liberal Culture and the Aesthetic.* Philadelphia: University of Pennsylvania Press, 2004.

Trollope, Anthony. *The Eustace Diamonds.* 1872. Oxford: Oxford University Press, 1998.

Turner, Bryan. *Citizenship and Capitalism.* London: Allen and Unwin, 1986.

Verdery, Katherine. "Whither 'Nation' and 'Nationalism'?" In *Mapping the Nation,* ed. Gopal Balakrishnan. New York: Verso, 1996. 226–34.

Vickery, Amanda. "Golden Age to Separate Spheres? A Review of the Categories and Chronology of English Women's History." *Historical Journal* 36.2 (1993): 383–418.

Wahrman, Dror. *Imagining the Middle Class: The Political Representation of Class in Britain, c. 1780–1840.* Cambridge: Cambridge University Press, 1995.

Walzer, Michael. "Citizenship." In *Political Innovation and Conceptual Change.* Cambridge: Cambridge University Press, 1989. 211–19.

———. "The Communitarian Critique of Liberalism." *Political Theory* 18.1 (February 1990): 6–23.

Williams, Raymond. *The Country and the City.* New York: Oxford University Press, 1973.

Wright, Kay Hetherly. "The Grotesque and Urban Chaos in *Bleak House.*" *Dickens Studies Annual: Essays on Victorian Fiction* 21 (1992): 97–112.

INDEX